A STROKE OF LUCK

On October 27, 1995, Dr. Howard Rocket suffered a massive stroke. A blood clot had lodged deep in his brain, several weeks following an accidental hit on the head during a pick-up football game.

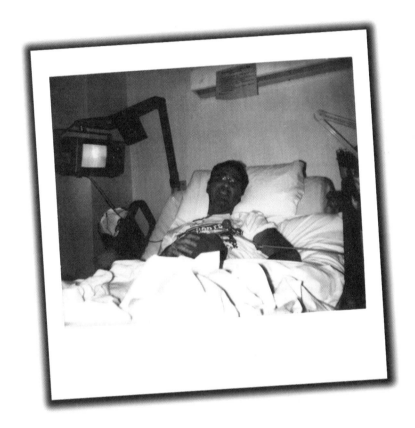

Howard came within hours of dying. He had been healthy, prosperous and successful—none of which mattered that day, because it was pure luck that saved Howard Rocket, along with heroic medical intervention by a team of dedicated specialists.

This book is the story of his life before the stroke, his brush with death, and his rebirth as a new person, in body and in spirit.

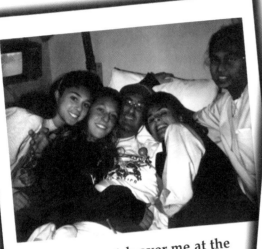

Family watch over me at the
Toronto Hospital, November 1995.

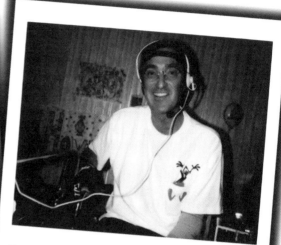

Positive attitude is the best medicine.

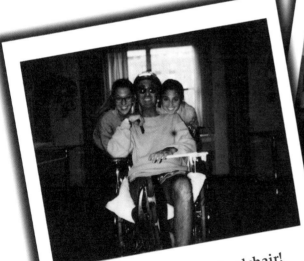

Rollerblades in my wheelchair!

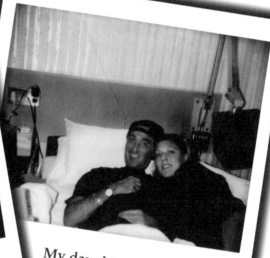

My daughter Dana with Dad.

"There was no way he was staying in this bed."
— from page 114

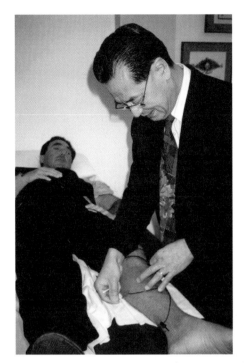
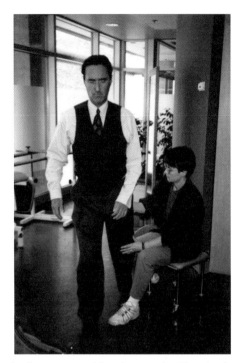

Acupuncture treatment, then extensive physiotherapy at Physio-Logic Physical Rehabilitation assisted in my recovery. Four months after the stroke, the Florida sun is a nice place to rest—my daughters are there to lend a hand.

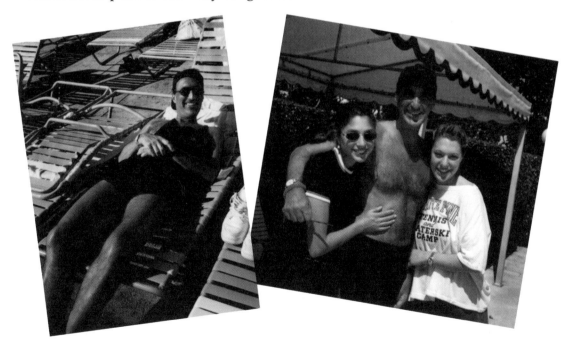

"He was alert and aware, and totally focused on recovery."
— from page 106

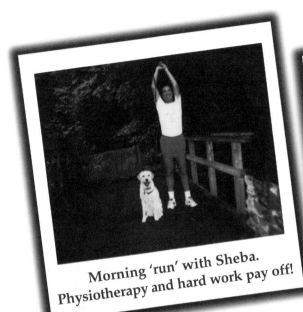

Morning 'run' with Sheba.
Physiotherapy and hard work pay off!

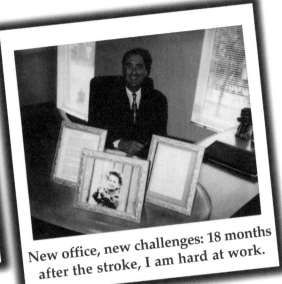

New office, new challenges: 18 months
after the stroke, I am hard at work.

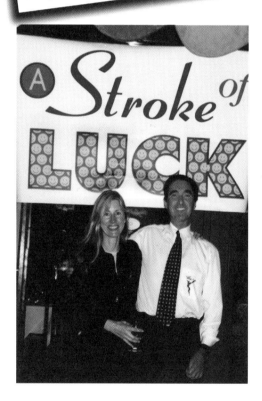

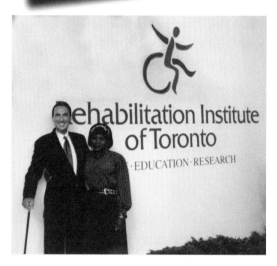

Nurse Glenda (above) welcomes me back
to Rehabilitation Institute of Toronto.
My friend and colleague, Jennifer Jackson,
and associates celebrate my return to work.

"... he'd survived ... and he was going to do everything else, too."
— from page 107

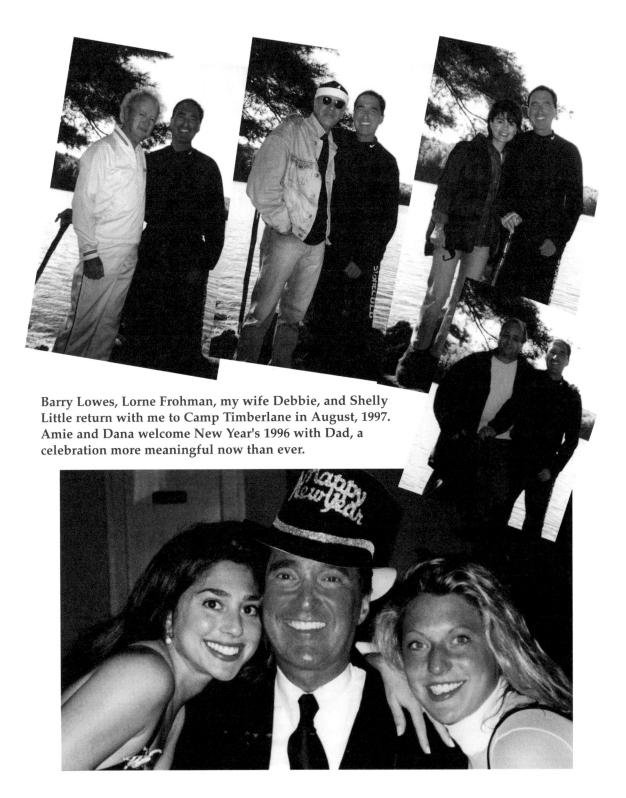

Barry Lowes, Lorne Frohman, my wife Debbie, and Shelly Little return with me to Camp Timberlane in August, 1997. Amie and Dana welcome New Year's 1996 with Dad, a celebration more meaningful now than ever.

"It certainly helped to have people around who cared ..."
— from page 85

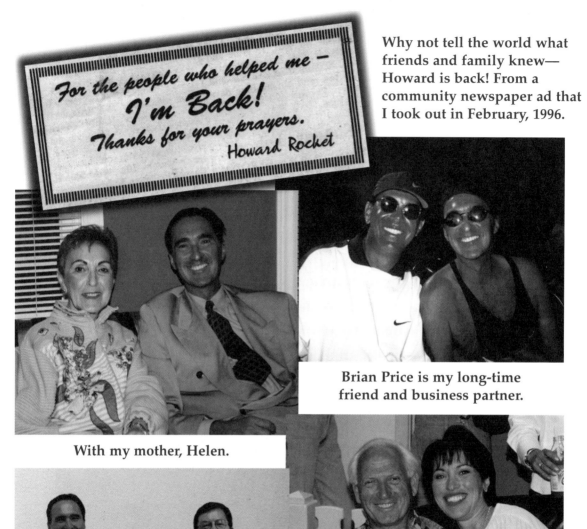

For the people who helped me —
I'm Back!
Thanks for your prayers.
Howard Rocket

Why not tell the world what friends and family knew—Howard is back! From a community newspaper ad that I took out in February, 1996.

Brian Price is my long-time friend and business partner.

With my mother, Helen.

My brother-in-law Sonny and sister Tyrral.

My good friend Kenny Field and I giving each other a hand.

"... they dealt with common tragedy by coming together."
— from page 84

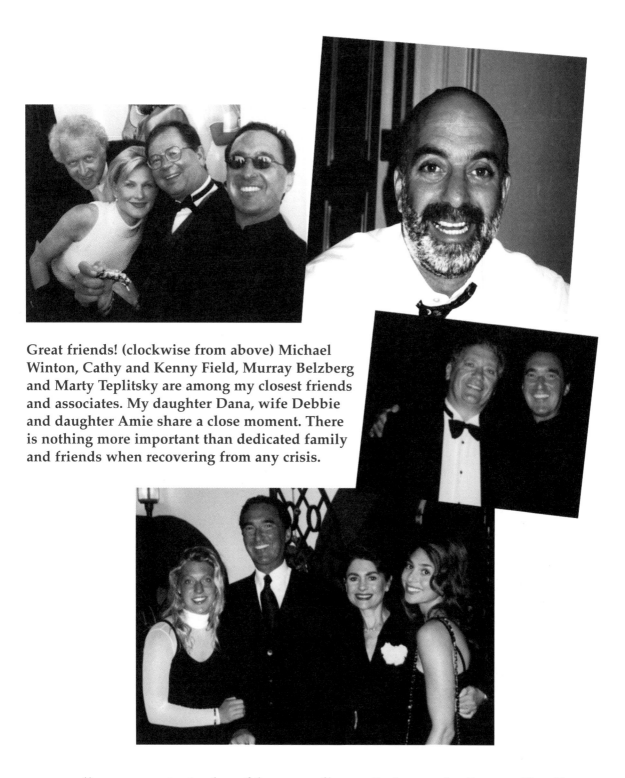

Great friends! (clockwise from above) Michael Winton, Cathy and Kenny Field, Murray Belzberg and Marty Teplitsky are among my closest friends and associates. My daughter Dana, wife Debbie and daughter Amie share a close moment. There is nothing more important than dedicated family and friends when recovering from any crisis.

"... a great circle of love ... flowed through them all ..."
— from page 173

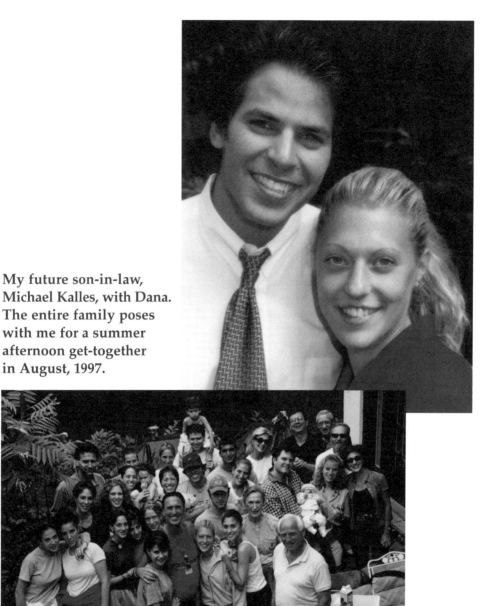

My future son-in-law,
Michael Kalles, with Dana.
The entire family poses
with me for a summer
afternoon get-together
in August, 1997.

*"Howard ... felt strongly the power of emotion and
devotion that linked each of these people together ..."*
— from page 179

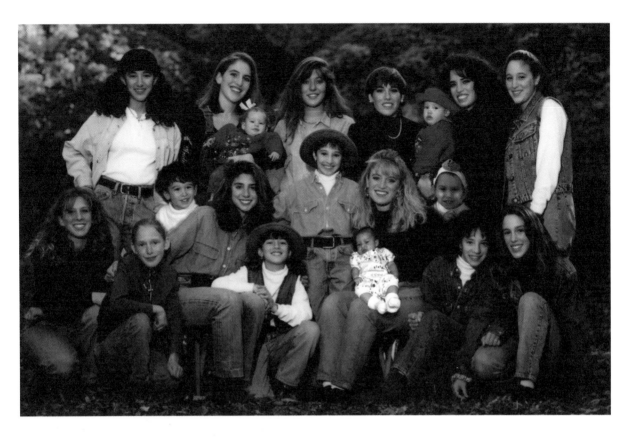

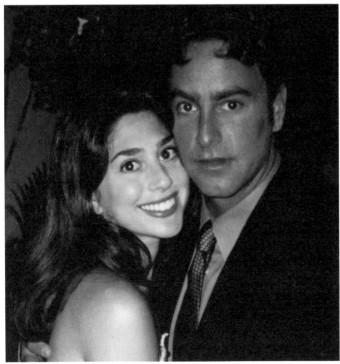

My beautiful nieces, devoted daughters, and only nephew on the Rocket side, Spencer, are a constant source of strength for me.

Michael Wuls, my son-in-law, with Amie. To witness their marriage in May, 1997 fulfilled a pledge I made when Amie was born.

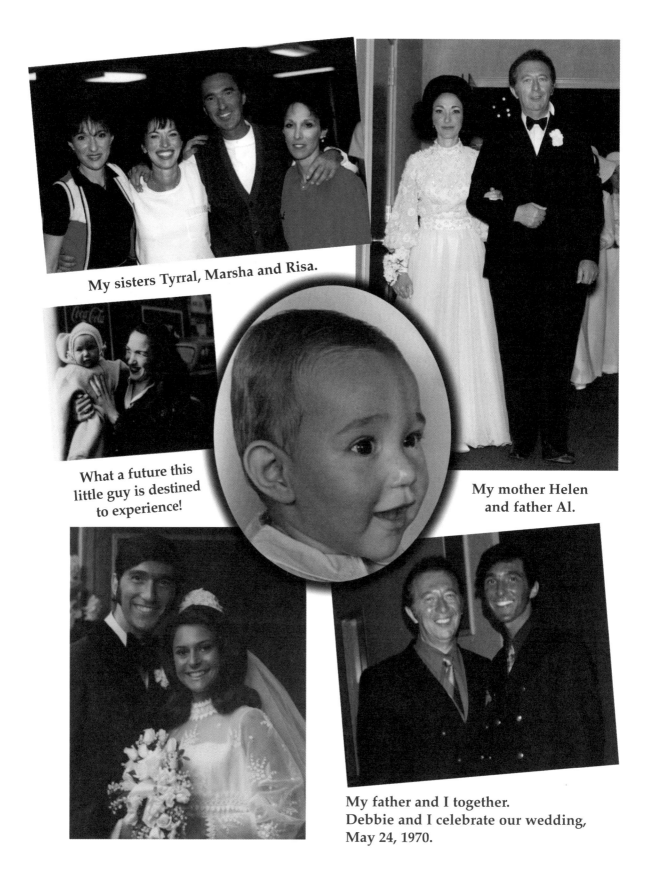

My sisters Tyrral, Marsha and Risa.

What a future this little guy is destined to experience!

My mother Helen and father Al.

My father and I together.
Debbie and I celebrate our wedding,
May 24, 1970.

life, crisis

and rebirth

of a stroke

survivor

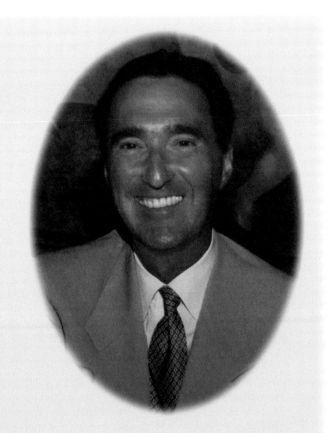

A STROKE OF LUCK

Dr. Howard Rocket

with Rachel Sklar

A Stroke of Luck
REVISED EDITION – Copyright ©1999 Toronto Rehabilitation Institute Foundation.
All Rights Reserved. No part of this book may be used or reproduced in any manner
whatsoever without written permission from the copyright holder, except in the case of
brief quotations embodied in news articles and book reviews.

Toronto Rehabilitation Institute Foundation
550 University Avenue, Toronto, Ontario, Canada M5G 2A2
Telephone: 416-597-3040 Fax: 416-597-6201 Web: http://www.rit.on.ca/

Published in association with Parnassus Communications & Publishing, Toronto
Telephone: 416-593-6993 Fax: 416-593-1173 E-Mail: books@planetcast.com

For bulk orders, special reprints and media inquiries, please contact:
Toronto Rehabilitation Institute Foundation
Telephone: 416-597-3040 Fax: 416-597-6201 E-Mail: foundation@rit.on.ca

Visit the special book web site featuring reader commentary, media archives,
and stroke information resources: http://www.StrokeOfLuck.com/

Book design by William C. Stratas / Parnassus Communications & Publishing.
Cover artwork by Dakis & Wilder Design Communications Inc.
Typesetting and page layout by WordsWorth Communications.
Web site design and hosting by Planetcast Presentations, Inc.
Printed in Canada.

Photography credits:
Jacket front: From the Rocket family album: Howard Rocket at a family
celebration on January 1st 1996, two months following his stroke.
Jacket inside back flap: Authors' photo by William C. Stratas.
Photo section, pages iii–xiii: From the Rocket family album.

This book was commissioned by Dr. Howard Rocket as a fundraising and awareness
tool for stroke research and prevention. One hundred percent of proceeds from sale
of this book go directly to stroke research, education and treatment.

Cataloguing in Publication Data

Rocket, Howard, 1947–
A stroke of luck: life, crisis, and rebirth of a stroke survivor

Revised Edition
ISBN 0-9696106-4-5

1. Rocket, Howard, 1947–   – Health. 2. Cerebrovascular disease – Patients –
Canada – Biography. I. Sklar, Rachel, 1972– . II. Title.

RC388.5.R625 1999   362.1'9681'0092   C98-933034-6

9 8 7 6 5 4 3 2

To Debbie, Amie, Dana,
the Michaels, ("The Man"), my wonderful
family, incredible friends, and all the
doctors and staff at the hospital:
I'll never forget you.

HOWARD ROCKET'S TREATMENT TIMELINE

Sunday September 17, 1995:
Howard Rocket accidentally hits his head on the ground while playing a pick-up football game with friends in a park. Throughout September and October he experiences moments of blurred vision and occasional pounding headaches. He is otherwise healthy, and expects that these symptoms will pass. They don't.

Friday October 27, 1995:
6:15 pm—Howard collapses in his bedroom, a violent explosion of searing pain ripping through his head. A blood clot had lodged in his brain, causing a stroke. **8:00 pm**—After initial emergency assessment, Howard enters the Intensive Care Unit and the stroke team rushes to his side.

Saturday October 28, 1995:
6:00 am—After careful analysis and electronic scanning of blood flow in Howard's brain, doctors decide to apply an experimental treatment by threading a drug catheter to the arterial blockage in his brain and injecting a clot-busting drug. **11:00 am**—Howard is out of immediate danger, but his condition is fragile. He is moved from the operating room to the neurological intensive care ward.

Tuesday October 31, 1995:
Howard wakes up and is aware of family and friends around him. The next day he is released from the ICU and moved to the recovery ward. By the end of November he is transferred to a rehabilitation hospital where he begins extensive physiotherapy and stroke recovery treatment.

January 1, 1996:
Howard 'walks' into the family's New Year's Day brunch, leaving his wheelchair in the car. Throughout 1996 he continues to make excellent progress. Eventually he resumes normal business and family activities.

August 1997:
Howard 'runs' up to 1/4 mile in the park. His cane is no longer needed. Although physiotherapy continues, his recovery is near completion.

The Major Warning Signs of Stroke

The following symptoms may indicate that a stroke is imminent. Medical attention must be sought as soon as possible after any of these warning signs are observed:

- Sudden weakness or numbness of the face, arm or leg, on one side of the body.

- Sudden dimness or loss of vision, particularly if it occurs in one eye.

- Loss of speech, or difficulty talking or understanding speech.

- Sudden, severe headaches with no apparent cause.

- Unexplained dizziness, unsteadiness, or sudden falls, especially when combined with any of the previous symptoms.

Source: The Canadian Family Guide to Stroke, page 37
Published by the Heart and Stroke Foundation of Canada, 1996

*This book was commissioned
by Dr. Howard Rocket as a
fundraising and awareness tool for
stroke research and prevention.*

*One hundred percent of proceeds from
sale of this book go directly to stroke
research, education and treatment.*

Contents

Your feedback on this book is welcomed. Comments for the authors may be left at our special web site, which features a discussion area for stroke survivors and families, plus other information in support of stroke prevention and education:

http://www.StrokeOfLuck.com/

Prologue

The human body isn't made to last. Eventually, something in the vast machine that carries us around every day of our life breaks down beyond repair. And when that is lost, we are lost; the whole cannot be whole without each of its parts.

I found that out the hard way. I almost died. But now I'm back.

And this is my story.

My story, like anyone and everyone else's. I am not unique. So why tell the story? Was my recovery extraordinary? Perhaps. Were the circumstances tragic? In some ways. But were they unique? No. I had a stroke, and then I recovered.

But that's not the story.

That's just what happened. The story isn't the what; it's the why, the who, the how. And it's precisely the fact that I'm *not* unique that makes this story worth telling.

Because what happened to me could happen to anyone, does happen—to anyone—every day. And if it hadn't happened to me I might have spent my entire life blind to what is important. Taking life for granted.

And that's not life. That's not even living.

I discovered that life is about more than success or wealth; I had all of that without realizing how much all my money was costing me. When my life was reduced to a few critical hours in the operating room, it wasn't Howard Rocket, entrepreneur and wheeler-dealer, who was lying on the table. It was Howie Rocket—father, husband, brother, son, friend. It was just me, just any guy—a rather unlucky guy who happened to have a tube in his brain.

But luck is defined by the moment, and at this moment I feel lucky indeed. Lucky to be alive. Lucky to have around me a warm circle of people whose support propelled me forward. Lucky to be able to savor the hard-won sweetness of moving a finger or taking a step. And, underlying all of these miracles, I am lucky to have had the stroke—without which all this amazing luck would have gone unnoticed.

People are shocked when I tell them that the stroke was the best thing that ever happened to me. My friends think about me lying wasted and gray in a hospital bed, unable to speak or see or move. My family thinks of the horror of losing me and how close they came to that horror. But I think of what my life was like before—or rather, what it *wasn't* like. Because it was missing a hell of a lot—and I didn't even know it! It was like thinking the moon is the brightest object in the sky because you've never seen the sun. But I've seen the sun now, and there's no way I'm going back. I know—I finally *know*—what's important in my life. I finally know.

If you're thinking that this is probably a book about re-evaluating priorities and not taking life for granted, you're right. If that doesn't interest you, stop reading. Go back to your daytimer and make sure you don't get off schedule. But I say that living out of a daytimer isn't living. And if it's living you're interested in, read on, because that's what this book is about.

It's about living, and loving, and learning. And I didn't do enough of all three before. But I never stop now.

But one doesn't do this in a vacuum. This story isn't mine alone. It belongs to every ripple that was caused when I plopped like a stone into a new kind of life. To those who lived and loved and learned themselves—for me, with me, and because of me.

That's not to say that this story is about happy endings all around. Grave situations can bring out the best in people—or the worst. And I have had my share of disappointments and betrayals. That's part of the learning. But then you slough off what has died, and it becomes part of the living. And if the ending isn't perfect, well, mostly perfect is still pretty damn good.

There's not much more to say about the story except to tell it. So here it is. It's a story about the family who stopped their lives to help mine start again. About the friends who stood by when nothing could be done, and in so doing did so much. About acquaintances who cared themselves into friends. About health care workers who perform everyday acts of heroism.

And it's about the extraordinary power of the ordinary person. In this case, it was me.

But it could be you.

—Howard Rocket

Beyond the Second Dimension

Apicture may be worth a thousand words, but often not the right ones—there's only so much that can be reflected from a two-dimensional plane. The camera captures only a microsecond of lives intertwined. A hastily arranged pose, a flash of sparkling teeth—who knows what lurks beneath the surface of the family photo?

In the Rocket family photos dated before October 27, 1995, the sparkly smiles are not much different from those taken later. But the thousand words evoked are. Because in later pictures, there are unseen elements that make their presence felt. A cane. A wheelchair. A hand that won't obey the brain that commands it. These are the constant reminders that separate what was from what is.

Reminders echo throughout the Rocket home, itself like any other, at least from the outside. Inside, every object has been invested with another dimension. The stairs that require an upright body to climb. The table that's too low for a wheelchair. The light switch that's too high. Just the everyday obstacles of your average, ordinary home.

But this is not your average, ordinary home. Because the bathroom has had a metal bar installed along the wall, and the living room was once arranged around a hospital bed. Not average, and not ordinary, but a home—home to the Rocket family and its own everyday images. Fresh-cut flowers on a tabletop, courtesy of Debbie. Photos of her daughters Amie and Dana, their own sparkly smiles befitting the dental hygiene of a dentist's kids. The dogs—Sheba, a frisky yellow lab pup and Humphrey, the sage, elderly Bijon-Frise who isn't about to yield an inch of his domain—tumbling over each other to greet whoever walks through the door. In this case, it's their master, Dr. Howard Rocket, who is striding in.

Striding? Is it possible that a man who is partially paralyzed on his left side could be striding?

Well, it depends how you define the word "striding." If you think it means walking purposefully with an even gait, with equal legs travelling with equal power over equal distances, then no, Howard Rocket does not stride. But if the word is evocative not so much of the movement as of what lies *behind* it, then there is no other word to describe the way Howard Rocket moves.

He strides in, giving Sheba and Humphrey their due, and slings his jacket off with one hand, his right hand. It's the hand he uses to knot his tie and his shoelaces, so a jacket is no problem. Time is precious to Howard, and he wastes little of it before settling his attention on some project or another. The phone rings. He has to take the call. He spends a few minutes dispensing decisive advice, puts the phone down, and is refocused.

Refocused. Howard had no choice but to refocus when his life was changed in an instant on Friday October 27, 1995. It was the day he suffered a massive stroke, the day he forever left the ease with which he'd taken for granted the smallest self-sufficiency, and realized the enormity of that smallness. Sure, Howard had had some headaches since he smacked his head during a pick-up football game weeks earlier, but who would have guessed that this superbly fit, healthy, vibrant, just-turned-forty-eight year old would be brought so low so fast? Certainly not Howard, whose pride in his physical fitness and healthy lifestyle was never in doubt. Not Howard, the dentist-cum-businessman who was too busy attending to the details of life to worry about any threat to it. Not Howard, just when business was going so great and he was on the cusp of even greater success. Not Howard. Who had time for a stroke?

But strokes can hit at the most inconvenient times, and this one didn't care that Howard didn't have it pencilled in. As strokes do, it exploded into his life without asking permission and took him on an unplanned journey, away from the life he had grown to believe was his. Dragging his world along with it. Momentarily erasing the sparkly smiles from the family snapshots.

One year later, and it's easy to forget. The sparkly smiles are back, and it's because Howard is back. The crisis has passed, life can go on, life does go on. Amie and Dana have their Dad back. Debbie no longer has to commute downstairs to the living room to tell her husband something in bed. Howard's back in business, meeting here, lunching there, focused and refocused. But the sparkly smiles reflect more now than just good dental hygiene—always important, mind you, but yes, there is more—they reflect relief, and awareness, and appreciation for the fact that a smile is still possible. And though Howard is back, he brought a lot back with him. The mark on his throat where a tube once passed through. The memory of what death felt like. The relief that he still knows what life feels like.

But it's a different kind of feeling—for everyone. Because Howard has changed, and that change is manifest in his relationships. In some ways it's a new Howard, someone who has learned and grown. But in some ways it's as though a time warp has brought back the Howard Rocket of yesteryear—a guy whose sisters, mom and buddies called "Howie." A guy who transformed slowly but unmistakably into "Howard" when he transformed suddenly and incredibly into an overnight success.

It's not that he turned into a calculating cutthroat. But when life sped up for Howard Rocket, something had to give. Across the board, a little time was sucked out, and he had to prioritize. No time to stop and smell the roses. Enter success. Exit reflection, meditation, contemplation, appreciation.

Smelling roses, smelling coffee, whatever. Howard smelled success and it was something he wanted more of. And why shouldn't he? He wasn't the type of person who could sit complacently on his laurels once a challenge had been surmounted. What world moved forward with that kind of attitude? Howard was a self-propelled forward-moving kind of guy. No place to go but up. And go on.

And up he went, taking his dreams and his bank balance with him. But he had to leave a little bit of himself behind; a smile here, a joke there; and he never really noticed it was gone, because there was so much else to marvel at, to relish, to discover. The trappings of success to sample. The limits of success to push.

And, of course, the benefits of success to share, with the family he loved more than anything. Nothing was spared for his gorgeous, growing daughters Amie and Dana, least of all his love, which he gave generously with lots more to spare. But he was always on the go, his mind was always a few steps ahead in his own personal mental marathon with no finish line. And he might have continued to run and run and run if he hadn't been forced to withdraw momentarily from the race.

Momentarily. Because running, striding, leaping and bounding are all still essential parts of Howard Rocket. Because running, striding, leaping and bounding are all functions of the will—and Howard has plenty of will. Just how much, he never quite knew, until he was forced to call upon hidden, dormant resources in order to accomplish the enormous tasks of sitting up in bed or swallowing a mouthful of food. Deep reserves of will of which he was unaware, back when he was unaware of much of his life. Was it his will that catapulted him from deathbed to striding cheerfully home to Sheba and Humphrey? Howard doesn't know. He only knows that breaking through walls means pushing the limits, again and again. It's how he believes he made his life—and how he got it back.

And how he'll keep it. Because every little self-sufficiency means freedom, means life. Taking a shower. Taking a step. Taking a breath. Howard knows now that these things come with deceptive ease, and it's something he's prepared to work hard for. And whenever someone tells him that it can't be done, he'll work twice as hard to prove them wrong. Just as he did when the doctors warned his family that he might never see again, or eat by himself, or write a letter, and don't even think about walking. Well, Howard did, and perhaps he thought himself out of his bed and onto his feet again.

Is there anything in modern medicine as potent as the will? Perhaps not, because medicine can only attend to the conglomeration of cells and atoms and molecules that we are, the stuff of life that we all come down to in the final analysis. But each of us is animated by something evasive, something that can't be predictably subdivided into the basic building blocks of matter—the soul, the other stuff of life. And it's from this stuff that the will comes. Though it can't be measured conventionally, it surfaces in acts like taking a shower, or a step, or a breath against all the odds.

For most of us, the mundane mechanisms of the human body pass unnoticed. But Howard notices now, and he's the first to point it out. How else can he unveil the worlds that are ignored every day? Expose all that is taken unwittingly for granted? Howard would say, "Hey, you. Reading this book. See, you're coming to the bottom of the page. You've got to turn it soon. Know how many muscles it takes to turn the page? Know how many muscles it takes to hold this book up?" And then, just as you turn the page, Howard's voice would continue: "I thought you didn't."

And that's all Howard really wants. To be the example you hope never to emulate, but still can learn from. To be a mirror reflecting life as it could be, as it should be. To be a billboard with WARNING! scrawled all over it in neon letters. To be an echo in your ear as you turn the page. To be the reminder of how hard the easiest things can be—and the illustration of how easy the hardest things can be. Without billboards, mirrors and echoes, the world overlooks its everyday miracles. Howard knows what that can lead to.

For him, it has led back home, among the fresh-cut flowers and the scampering dogs, the frantic phone calls and the cutting-edge projects. Back to the life he thought he'd lost, and to a life he never thought to find. Ultimately, it has led him back to his rightful place within the family snapshots. And as the shutter clicks, the moment is again complete, and so, finally, is the picture.

With sparkly smiles intact.

Just Another Life Story

When Howard Rocket was eighteen, he played Ponty Finch in the musical *How To Succeed in Business Without Really Trying*. Finch is a young whippersnapper who claws his way up the corporate ladder by dint of determination, opportunism, ingenuity and sheer drive. Howard was a young whippersnapper. But what the audience didn't realize was that they were being invited to take a peek into the future, when the role would be played for real in the drama called Howard's life. Because the casting was prophetic; Howard Rocket would indeed succeed. By dint of determination, opportunism, ingenuity and sheer drive.

To those who knew him, that was apparent from the start. As big brother to Marsha and Risa, Howie was accustomed to taking a leadership role—when his older sister Tyrral would let him. While Howie could get away with teasing the younger girls—especially Marsha—mercilessly, he had to fight tooth and nail to compensate for those three crucial years Tyrral had on him. Between poor victimized Marsha and the constant brawling of her two eldest, Helen Rocket had her hands full. Wasn't it enough that she had to make do for a family of six? Her husband Al made a decent living for his family, but selling life insurance was by no means a ticket to the big-time back in the 1950s, and Helen had learned early to make a buck go a long way. A regimented and relentlessly efficient woman,

Helen kept her family in line by demanding an environment of cleanliness and order. At the Rocket dinner table the plates were passed around in neat, carefully measured portions calculated for nourishing but not necessarily for noshing. Having to stretch their dollars meant frugality over frivolity. Perhaps foreshadowing future Rocket entrepreneurs, Helen became a competent, effective manager, culling from inner resources of strength and smarts the ability to run a tight ship—as long as everyone was on a tight leash.

With such a resource to fall back on, Al Rocket could lapse into his easygoing nature after putting in his hours offering insurance to those prudent and willing enough to oblige. The second-generation son of Polish immigrants, Al was the only Rocket out of seven children; the original "Rocketovitz" had been shortened by well-meaning immigration officers to Rocket, which Al's younger siblings had abjured in favor of 'Rockert.' Al was happy enough to keep what Canadian immigration had bestowed. The only boy, Howie alone could carry on that lone family name.

Being the only boy had its advantages. A skinny, happy-go-lucky kid with an enterprising sense of humor, Howie was behind many a practical joke that would inevitably torment his sisters and exasperate his mother. But Howie was so good-humored that Helen's exasperation would soon be overtaken by her appreciation and affection for her wacky, energetic son. That would be enough to tide Howie over until the next prank.

These advantages aside, Howie still yearned for a brother. His hopes were vested briefly in the baby that was born five years after him, but when it turned out to be just another girl, those hopes were crushed. Poor five-year-old Howie was not pleased, and manifested his extreme disappointment as five-year-old boys do—in a ferocious tantrum complete with kicking and screaming. Alas, Howie's behavior was not enough to magically transform a Marsha into a Marshall. He had to adapt to his fate. As luck would have it, five-year-olds are extremely adaptable, and he was no exception. Besides, there were benefits to having a younger sister, like teasing and bossing privileges, of which Howie made good use. Nine years later along came Risa, and Howie was firmly established in the role of big brother.

Not that Howie wanted for male companionship. The Little family, who lived across the street from the Rocket home on Castlewood Avenue, had their own handful, who went by the name of Shelly. Born a few months apart, Shelly and Howie grew up together. They were classmates through grammar and high school and remained together all the way to Dentistry at the University of Toronto. In fact, the two encountered the myriad possibilities of dentistry early on. Shelly, never a little person, took it upon himself to jump on young Howie's back in the yard of Allenby Public School. Slight Howie couldn't quite hold up under his friend's weight, and was thrown forward—teeth first—into the brick building. The caps on his two front teeth now bear proud witness to that fateful day—as do the careers of both roughhousers.

Howie had to wait a long time for a brother, but he finally found one in Sonny Prashker, Tyrral's boyfriend. Howie, newly Bar-Mitzvahed and growing fast, relished the prospect of an instant older brother and took to Sonny immediately. The fact that Sonny eventually married Tyrral and took her out of the house was even better—now Howie was the oldest and truly the boss. But by that time he was more interested in success in sports and school than in harassing his younger sisters, although he always kept some teasing in reserve for special occasions.

Howie also had his father for male companionship. Howie loved Al fiercely, looking to him for approval and encouragement. While Helen was the strong-willed woman of mettle, Al was the gentle, amiable rock of Howie's formative years. Howie devoted his inexhaustible energies to achieving for his parents, promising them grandly that he'd grow up, buy them a Cadillac convertible, and take care of them forever. He loved his parents. It was a promise he took seriously.

And it was a promise that looked like it might just be fulfilled. Ever the entrepreneur, Howie was always devising new methods of doing this or alternatives to doing that. If there was an inconvenience or inefficiency in life, Howie would nose it out and do his damnedest to correct it. When he was about fifteen, he came pretty close. At that time, milk was sold in three-quart jugs with a centered spout. During Friday night dinners with the family, Howie found out the hard way that these jugs were a pain in the neck. Every Friday the family would sit down to Helen's meticulously prepared evening meal. Every Friday they'd finish dinner and serve tea and coffee. And every Friday Howie would try to pour the milk, and would succeed only in generously splashing it across his mother's clean and ordered table. Every Friday, Helen would not be pleased.

Howie wasn't pleased, either. For a person who craved success, being a hopeless failure at pouring milk irked him considerably. After weeks of repeating the same mistake, Howie concluded that the problem lay not with him but with the milk jug. Within a few days, Howie had invented a three-quart jug that he believed to be spillproof. His idea was simple, as most good ones are: he had devised a jug with an off-center spout. This would revolutionize how milk was poured, for instead of tilting the jug at extreme angles, causing the fluid to rush out uncontrollably, the milk could be poured by allowing the container to rest on the flat side of the container. He showed it to Sonny, and was vindicated: Sonny thought it an ingenious invention and was immediately galvanized to market the jug. Howie's career as an entrepreneur was about to take off.

Sonny and Howie had a prototype made out of acrylic. They took it to Borden's Dairy, and were rewarded by real enthusiasm and, better yet, real interest: Borden's wanted the jug. Howie's invention was a success. Or it would have been a success if Borden's hadn't called back and regretfully declined because of a small but hope-dashing detail: all of Borden's containers were washed before being filled—and all their washing equipment was designed for center spouts. Howie learned early that efficiency can often run counter to practicality. Years later, when off-center spouts began appearing on oil containers and water bottles, Howie would have the satisfaction of knowing he had been onto something good. Of course, he wouldn't have the satisfaction of a patent, but he could live with that.

Meanwhile, there was still the business of getting through adolescence—no mean feat for a growing boy. An athletic, ambitious teenager, Howie's natural appetite for conquest became focused, a laser-intense beam that he directed full-force into his latest challenge. Whatever he undertook, he wanted to be good at—no, great at—and he would work until he excelled. Such was the case with tennis, his first love of sport, which he discovered long before it became fashionable. Howie stroked many a ball and smashed many a serve to ascend the levels of proficiency and eventually become a junior champion. Having attained the mastery he sought, Howie was satisfied, and turned his attention toward newer heights to scale.

Like making money. Burning up the courts was fun, but it wouldn't pay for the expenses of a burgeoning teenager in the early sixties. Howie knew better than to ask Helen for spending money. If he wanted anything, he learned to work for it. And work he did, at any odd job he could pick up. He worked for his father's younger brother Art (one of the Rockert clan) at his pizzeria, twirling dough or piling on toppings or doing whatever needed to be done. Anything to make a buck, he'd work for the post office delivering parcels, displaying his entrepreneurial flair by hiring a little kid to go up the steps with the parcels so he didn't have to. He worked at Town Shoes in Yorkdale Shopping Centre, bending low with shoe after shoe for foot after foot, day after day. Between his odd jobs, Howie scraped together just enough to support his adolescent lifestyle. Besides, he knew he could always hit up Sonny for a loan if he needed one, and the Prashker vehicles were always made available for Howie's romantic excursions.

Sonny also gave him steady work over the summers, employing Howie in his embroidery factory as a machine helper in maintaining the textile looms that ground away around the clock. It was this experience that solidified Howie's vague, overarching ambitions into the cold, clear realization that there was nothing for him to fall back on. Day after day in the factory taught Howie something that deep down he knew already: he wasn't interested in menial work. He wasn't interested in punching the clock. He wasn't interested in scraping by, stretching dollars, portioning meals, scrounging jobs. He wanted to achieve and to excel, and to be his own boss. To buy his parents a Cadillac. To buy *himself* a Cadillac. And he couldn't do that with his hands. He had to do it with his brain.

But in the meantime, Howie was doing all right for himself as teenagers went. He had his own money and the independence that came with it. He had a constant sense of humor, two hapless younger sisters to unleash it on, and his whole life ahead of him. He was open to new experiences. Which is why, when his old friend Shelly Little called him up one August and told him about an opening on the tennis staff at Camp Timberlane, Howie decided that it might be fun to try something new. So Howie picked up mid-summer and headed off to greet whatever camp had in store for him. As it turned out, it was a pretty good decision.

He arrived up at Timberlane and was met by Shelly, who was a veteran camper. Together, they walked up the tree-lined camp road into main camp and Howie took in the scenery. Walking down the camp road in the other direction was fifteen-year-old Debbie Kritzer. Howie took in that scenery, too. He turned to Shelly.

"She's going to be my girlfriend for the summer," he said matter-of-factly. Shelly snorted. Debbie Kritzer was, hands down, the best-looking girl in camp. Everyone wanted her. But beautiful Debbie Kritzer was still young, in no hurry, and was quite discriminating about whom she spent her much sought-after time with.

"Good luck with Frigid Bridget," he said, laughing at his skinny, determined friend.

Other male staff had the same reaction as Shelly. All they saw was this new kid, all legs and nose and teeth and abundant self-confidence, breezing into camp halfway through and planning to waltz off with the most sought-after girl under the Timberlane sun. Ludicrous! Impossible! But Howie didn't believe in the word impossible; every milk jug had to have its off-center spout.

So Howie set out to find it, between teaching tennis and enjoying the athletic, energetic freedom that is summer camp.

Auditions for the camp play eventually rolled around. It was *How To Succeed in Business Without Really Trying*, and its director was Lorne Frohman, one of Howie's new buddies, who, like most, thought his romantic aspirations a tad unrealistic. He also found out that Howie had artistic aspirations that were equally improbable when Howie announced his intention to win the leading role of J. Pierpont Finch—made even more improbable because it was the role that Lorne himself wanted. And, as director, it was his role to cast. Besides, he was dubious about the ability of this earnest, energetic, enterprising guy to play the role of an ambitious up-and-comer convincingly. Little did he know. And who knew if he could sing? Dance? Who was this little upstart from Toronto, anyway? But he was struck by Howie's sheer positive energy, his absolute conviction and confidence, and his upbeat attitude. Lorne finally was worn down by the utter totality of Howie's determination. The laser beam of Howie's drive was focused. What could he do? Howie would play Ponty Finch.

Naturally, the leading female role of Rosemary, a lovely, charming ingenue, could go to none other than Debbie Kritzer. Which, of course, was no surprise to Howie—he'd found his off-center spout and this time there would be no spilled milk. So there was Howie on stage, clawing and catapulting his way to the top of the heap, singing to himself an anthem of self-confidence called "I Believe in You." And there was Debbie, looking at this fiercely driven young man and realizing that there could be no other match for her. And there was Lorne, mouth gaping open on the sidelines in disbelief—this guy was actually good! And, finally, there were all the other guys—including Shelly—equally stunned, because Howie had done what he said he would do: he won the heart of the untouchable, unattainable, Debbie Kritzer. Life had imitated art. Howie was the only one who wasn't surprised. After all, he'd said he was going to do it, so what was the big deal?

He dismissed it from his mind. After all, there were more challenges out there.

An Ascending Path

The next few years passed like a blur for Howie, defined by one direction—up. Howie knew what he wanted—success. And the manifestation of success—money. With these entwined goals firmly in sight, Howard Rocket moved decisively from boyhood to manhood in the pursuit of the life he would claim as his own.

His experience in Sonny's factory had taught him well to rely on his brain in making that claim. The laser beam was now focused on the future, and the present was focused on making that future possible. Through pizza flipping, parcel delivering and shoe selling, Howie quietly accumulated enough money to take his education one step further. Thriving at the University of Toronto, he settled on dentistry as a sound career choice. Armed with self-confidence, ability, drive and a very respectable set of teeth, Howie set out to excel and achieve. It was important to achieve. It was important to be a success, to prove and be proven. It was more than important. It was everything.

Well, not quite everything. As goal-oriented and focused as Howie was, he was still human. And though he did his utmost to cultivate his brain, there was still the issue of his heart. Debbie Kritzer had first captured it on a sunny Timberlane path, and her hold upon it had remained firm. Ever since that summer, Howie and Debbie commuted between Toronto and Hamilton. Time went on, the commute became more regular, and somewhere along the line Debbie Kritzer became Debbie Rocket and life became truly whole.

By this time Howard was preparing to launch himself into the world of dentistry and to unleash his creative energy on the unsuspecting mouths of his patients. But Howie didn't want just any practice. Always mindful of his goal to innovate, excel and achieve, Howie established a joint practice with his colleague Shelly Bleiman and a young doctor by the name of Rick Sheppard. They founded a medical-dental center with a marketing twist designed to double their client base.

It worked. Slowly but surely, the center attracted a steady stream of customers who were willing to submit to Howie's dental machinations. Proficiency in his chosen craft was important to Howie, but achieving that was not enough. He wanted to be not just a good dentist but a *fast* one. Working with speed and efficiency was inextricably linked with Howie's notion of good dentistry, and he developed a deft dental touch that quickened his pace without compromising his handiwork.

Howie's hands weren't the only things moving swiftly. In a few years Howie had married, graduated and built the life he knew was his. Barely a year after starting his practice, Debbie gave birth to a beautiful baby girl they named Amie. Two fleeting years later she was followed by little Dana. And suddenly there was Howie—father, husband, man of the house, provider for his family. Getting by was no longer as easy as borrowing the car from Sonny or flipping pizza dough for Uncle Art. Howie was standing on his own. There was no more Helen to neatly apportion meals and keep the ship tight. No more Risa and Marsha to terrorize offhandedly.

And suddenly, no more Al. The sturdy foundation of Howie's childhood, the quiet backbone of his life, his father, gone. Al had been diagnosed with an auto-immune blood disorder that struck quickly, leaving behind a bewildered family grieving for the centerpiece of their existence. All eyes turned to Howie to shoulder the mantle left vacant by the loss of Al. He had no choice. The last Rocket male became head of the Rocket family. He was twenty-seven.

It wasn't easy, but Howie didn't need easy to get by. Life had too many responsibilities to waste time on complaints. Howie had two growing daughters, one wildly growing practice, and his entire family to maintain and secure. Tyrral, Sonny and their family were doing fine, thank God, but Marsha was twenty-two and had only just gotten married. And Risa was still a kid, barely seventeen. She still needed a big brother. And Helen—well, Helen needed someone to take care of her so she could take care of everybody else. Howie knew what he had to do. He owed it to his family. He owed it to his father.

So Howie became all things to all people as his daughters blossomed before his eyes and his life continued steadily upon the path he'd sworn himself to take so long ago. Self-sufficient, prosperous, secure and established, Howie was standing on his own. Which he loved. Which had been his goal. Which he'd worked hard as hell to achieve. Which he had never doubted for a moment would come to pass.

Yet still something was missing, and it didn't take Howie long to figure out what it was. Thrilled as he was with his success, he wanted more. It wasn't enough to be a good, even a great dentist, to extract a molar quickly and cleanly with still more molars lined up at the door. It just wasn't enough. He'd been at it for almost a decade, and no longer got a charge out of drilling, filling and scraping plaque. He wanted more, much more.

For Howie, goals achieved yielded only to further goals. He thought, *I'm married, I have a family, I have a home, I*

*have success, I have stability, I have money. I have the perfect
life. So where do I go from here?* Howie was bored. He wanted
to use his brain, tackle problems, forge solutions, mold answers. He knew there were an infinite number of off-center
spouts out there waiting to be discovered.

And it wasn't long before he found one.

Howard Rocket saw a need in the dental profession. It
was a need for more people like him—fast, efficient, customer-
oriented. He had built his practice on speed and efficiency.
Why not take what he'd learned and apply it on a grand scale?
He saw a chance to improve how dental offices operated and
how patients were served. Dentistry had been dominated by
nine-to-five offices with little flexibility and even less efficiency. But patients took what they could get. They had no
choice. Howie wanted to give them a choice, and he was confident they'd choose him.

The concept was simple: store-front dentistry. Howie would
take dentistry to the people en masse, promising service, value
and convenience. Howie recognized that patients were also
customers operating in a free market, and he wanted them to
feel free to come to him. A chain of clinics would offer dental
access from numerous locations, all under one recognizable
name that would quickly become a familiar sight in shopping
malls and plazas: Tridont Dental Centres.

Tridont. So named for the trio of dentists who brought the
concept to life—Howie, his partner Shelly, and another class-
mate named Brian Price. Well, it began as a trio, but Shelly
decided early on to opt out and left the project, with his blessing, to Brian and Howie. From Tridont to ... Duodont? No way,
they liked the original name. So they kept it. If things went
well soon they'd have a lot more than three dentists working
for them.

Things went well. Suddenly Howie was no longer bored—the laser had locked onto something and there was no time for his mind to stray. Because his mind was busy—incredibly busy, planning and exploring and implementing and creating this wonderful new enterprise with which to attract the dentist-going population. Howie rejoiced in his brain's perpetual activity. His spirit delighted in the thrill of this new challenge, and his bank account celebrated by swelling obligingly. Dentistry was fun!

Anything's fun when you're sitting on top of the world, and Howie and Brian certainly were. Their idea took off like a shot, breathing life into a profession that had, without innovation, grown somewhat stale. Customers loved it. Other dentists hated it. Resistant to change and resentful of being prodded to accept it, the dental community took a palpable dislike to Howie, Brian and their merry band of obliging dentists under the friendly and welcoming Tridont umbrella. Dentists, so comfortable for so long in the tacitly upheld oligopoly of their craft, were suddenly being challenged. Who were these upstart guys, opening extended hours, occupying mall space between the food court and the jeans store? Dentistry didn't much like these young mavericks—even if the public did.

As usual, Howie didn't care. He was too busy lapping up the dazzling bounty of success. My God, having money could be fun! The part of Howie that was still a kid loved the toys available to him—the flashy cars, the sophisticated electronic gadgetry, the clothes—all the *stuff*. He loved stuff. He loved *owning* stuff. The part of Howie that remembered portioned meals took a fierce joy in lavishing everything on Debbie, Amie and Dana, and others he loved. He moved his family out of their townhouse—purchased once upon a time because it was across the street from Shelly Little and his family—and settled in a deluxe bungalow on an upscale street. He presented his mother with a convertible, making good on a promise he made to his parents long ago. He loved his parents. It was a promise he took seriously.

Howie was on top of the world. He had done it! He had used his brain to propel him to heights he had dreamed of as a kid. Pretty good for a guy who wasn't even close to approaching his forties. And it wasn't only the money and the notoriety and the respect that did it for him either, although that was pretty damn good. It was the fact that it was all because he had *created* something new, improved the world in some small way, made it *better*. Millions of sparkly toothed customers couldn't be wrong, which meant that Howie had done something right.

And not just with his hands, either. He'd teamed up with a colleague just like him, a dreamer and a go-getter, and together they'd made it work. Now they paid other people to hold the drill and apply the fluoride, because they were too busy running the business behind the drill. Dealing with the everyday crises of a dynamic, expanding, thriving business. Tackling problems, forging solutions, molding answers. Howard wasn't just a dentist, he was a *businessman*, an *entrepreneur*. People knew who he was and what he'd done; the name Dr. Howard Rocket *meant* something. He'd arrived, dammit. Howard Rocket had arrived. And he loved every second of his new life.

He loved being rich. He loved being successful. He loved seeing his children grow up with every opportunity. He loved seeing his beautiful wife in a beautiful home wearing beautiful clothes. He loved wheeling and dealing, taking phone calls and meetings, driving through the city wearing shades and a smile, or being driven by his chauffeur when he was too busy to drive. He loved spending weekends at his beautiful cottage when his schedule allowed and spending money on frivolous pleasures without thinking about it. And he loved that he had done it all on his own, creating it from next to nothing, bringing it forth from pizza dough flipped and parcels delivered and shoes sold.

It was a good thing he loved it, because it occupied most of his time. Not that he didn't have time to watch Amie and Dana grow more gorgeous every day—his family came first. But the laser was out in full force and once focused, didn't appreciate being scattered. Between the meetings, faxes and phone calls, Tridont kept growing and Howard had to keep up. There was always more to do and explore and accomplish, and the limits to push kept expanding with the scope of his business vision and ambition.

But pushing the limits had its drawbacks, too. Resistant to and resentful of change, the dental profession watched Howard and Brian guardedly. Dentistry is a self-governing profession, with its own standards and rules, conservative and established and entrenched. Pushing the limits meant hovering dangerously close to the line, and there were a lot of people watching, just waiting for that line to be crossed.

It was only a matter of time, really. Howard and Brian's approach to dentistry was as a business. And, like any business, it had to be marketed. Howard and Brian would have happily spent money on large-scale ad campaigns, but the profession was strictly regulated, with definite rules against overt advertising. The Royal College of Dental Surgeons only allowed the publication of a practitioners business card. The Tridont boys got around that detail by taking out a full-page ad in the major papers—composed entirely of business cards, one for each new Tridont dentist. Technically within the rules, but definitely pushing the limits. Other dentists complained. The College took notice. People were watching even more closely.

But Howard and Brian kept pushing the envelope—until the envelope ripped. Emboldened by their marketing coup, they agreed to appear in magazine ads endorsing Holiday Inns of Canada. Billed as "new faces of the Canadian establishment," the ads showed the busy and successful Drs. Rocket and Price of Tridont Dental Centres, working and building and creating, and staying at Holiday Inn, which met all their travel needs. Howard and Brian, confident and sure, smiling in agreement from the double-page spread.

All hell broke loose. Finally, those dentists who had been the bitterest about Tridont and its troublesome founders had their *own* off-center spout. More than a few detailed complaints were registered with the College, and Howard and Brian found themselves facing disciplinary action for acting in breach of regulations, charged with professional misconduct.

Howard and Brian were incensed. They knew the rules and abided by them. This wasn't about paying a fine or taking a slap on the wrist. Just because no one else had done it before didn't make it wrong! They had succeeded, it was as simple as that. If the profession didn't like it, fine. But it was *their* success, and damned if they weren't going to use it as they pleased.

They didn't even bother defending the charge at the College level—they knew where that would lead them. Instead, they went straight to court, bringing a challenge under the *Canadian Charter of Rights and Freedoms*, at that time a relatively young and uninterpreted statute. They claimed that their right to freedom of expression, guaranteed in the *Charter* under section 2(b), had been violated by the College and thus by the provincial government, which had passed the College's governing act. They asserted that commercial expression was a fundamental right protected under the *Charter*, and implored the court to find in their favor.

Early Charter interpretation in Ontario courts was extremely conservative, so they had no chance of success. The court ruled against Howard and Brian. More than a few dentists were smug. But Howard wasn't fazed. He didn't recall ever having taken 'no' for an answer. Hell, he'd landed Debbie Kritzer at Timberlane! Other challenges paled in comparison. He and Brian took their case to the Ontario Court of Appeal, hoping that their plight, as presented by winning legal raconteur Marty Teplitsky, would move the court to overturn the lower judgment. But despite Marty's inspired arguments, the Court of Appeal denied their appeal in a 2-1 split. Howard looked at Brian. Brian looked at Howard. They both looked at Marty. And smiled. They had come this far, they might as well go all the way. And so Howard and Brian took their case to the Supreme Court of Canada, hoping to change the law that governed the nation.

It was a landmark case. Now the legal community joined the nation's dentists in watching Howard and Brian. Whatever the outcome, it would set the parameters for the right to freedom of expression in Canada. Whether those parameters included commercial expression was the question. Howard and Brian knew they were fighting now for more than just the chance to hock hotel rooms. It was a question of fundamental freedom for all Canadians, and what limits could justifiably be placed on those freedoms. They'd both fought for a lot in their lives, but never for anything quite on this scale. It was out of their hands now. Whatever the defining legal minds of the land decided, would become the law. It was that simple.

It was, it turned out, even simpler. The court was unanimous: Howard and Brian were right. Their right to freedom of expression under the *Canadian Charter of Rights and Freedoms* had indeed been violated. The regulation forbidding them to advertise was null and void. Their unblemished professional records were restored. Tridont right, College wrong. Case closed. They had won.

They had won! They had fought the battle for Tridont and had won it for businesses across the nation. They had pushed the limits again, expanding the rights of Canadians and making new law. This one was on the books. They'd made dental *and* legal history. Their smug dental adversaries weren't smiling anymore, although soon they too would realize what a favor had been done for them by those guys at Tridont.

Those guys at Tridont had indeed done them good, by yet again reshaping the way the dental profession operated in Canada. But the profession had undergone its own profound reshaping since the case had begun. That was four busy, hectic, whirling years before, and so much had happened since then. Howard had learned a lot in those frenzied four years that spun past him so swiftly he barely had time to notice himself turn forty.

That might have been because he was still gulping challenges like a twenty-year-old, or it might have been because he had far too much to think and worry about. Whatever the reason, Howard and Brian may have won at the Supreme Court, but it was something of a Pyrrhic victory because Tridont was in trouble.

It didn't seem that way at the beginning. In fact, things couldn't have been better. Tridont was thriving, Howard and Brian were rich, and teeth across Canada were better for it. Everybody was happy. But why not be happier? This was Howard, and leaving well enough alone was not his strong suit. Howard and Brian had thought about it, and decided that it was time to take Tridont public. Their success to that point was considerable, but it paled in comparison to the heights to which they could soar with public investment. Bigger and better was just around the corner.

So Tridont went public on the Toronto Stock Exchange. And the public went to Tridont. Howard and Brian traded total ownership and control for the money pouring into the Tridont treasury, representing the potential for even more success and innovation. Because if Tridont had worked so well for dentistry, there must be thousands of possible applications for their concept! The possibilities were limited only to their ideas. And their ideas weren't limited at all. Pretty soon Howard and Brian had expanded the Tridont business model to areas as diverse as optical centres, footcare, and nursing homes. The brokers were happy—the capital was invested, the stock was moving. The practitioner/shareholders were happy—they were making money, so far. Howard and Brian were happy—their stellar success story kept advancing.

Yes, everyone was happy—until things started sliding. Howard and Brian had expanded rapidly into uncharted waters, and that error in judgment was becoming apparent. Unlike the original Tridont Dental Centres, which were predicated on their professional training, these new businesses went beyond Howard and Brian's area of expertise—into retail optical, chiropractic, and foot care. Howard and Brian knew teeth. More to the point, they knew the business of teeth, which was important. But they were unfamiliar with the business of their growing business, which divested them of critical autonomy and control and made them reliant on advisers and managers. The only profitable business was the dental division—it was very profitable, but was it profitable enough to prop up the entire enterprise?

Ultimately, it was not. Successful though they were, Howard and Brian were not successful enough to offset the losses generated by the new endeavors.

Tridont went into receivership and no one involved was happy. Not the brokers, who had encouraged investors to place their bets with Tridont. Not the Tridont practitioners, many of whom had invested their own money in Tridont stock, confident in the precedent of success set by Howard and Brian. And not Howard and Brian, who had been twice as confident about the empire they had built from the ground up. Especially not Howard and Brian, who watched their empire skidding out of control and felt themselves powerless to stop it.

The years of building, growing, watching ideas take shape—all gone. It was amazing how it all could skid out of grasp. Did Howard feel like a failure? No way. Because by that time Tridont dentists knew the drill. They understood that a profitable, efficient dental practice wasn't only about using their hands. Tridont had been the agent of change as dentists recognized the need to run their practices as businesses, and treat patients as customers.

Did Howard think himself a failure? No way. Because as defunct as Tridont itself may have been, the concept remained valid. And it was the concept that was important. Howard Rocket and Brian Price left a legacy that would endure to this day. Storefront dentistry was the way of the future, and it had been *their* way first. *They* had pioneered the notion of dentist-as-businessman. *They* had changed the standards of the profession and met the expectations of customers. *They* had widened the scope of professional freedom. *They* had broken down walls and leapt over barriers.

And as far as Howard was concerned, that was what really mattered.

Pinnacle

Tridont was over. But life wasn't, and that meant finding something else to do. Howard had no problem with that, he'd been doing it all his life. And there were innumerable opportunities, infinite directions in which to move from where he stood, poised to take on anything. Working without Tridont meant being totally free. How many people get that lucky in the prime of their careers?

Being free meant having choices. And Howard had already made one: he was never going back to practising dentistry. He'd closed that door firmly. He'd gotten a taste of being in business, and he liked it. He was creative, he was aggressive. How creative could you be with a root canal? You get aggressive with a drill and before you know it you're in court. No, Howard's involvement in the dental profession would be strictly limited to business.

But before he could leap into the future, he had to extricate himself from the past. The business shell of Tridont Health Care had to be wound down. Howard was trapped in limbo between exciting ventures, and mired in the mundane, detail-oriented present. Details! Ugh. Howard hated them. The laser chafed uncomfortably. His brain itched to *do* something.

What could he do? He was a slave to the laser. His creativity took hold. So he painted. He spent days, nights, months, just painting, releasing his mental energy, his hands a fury of brushwork, pouring the images from his brain onto canvas after canvas. His makeshift studio became the headquarters of his intellectual aggression, the place where he could make something that hadn't been there before. So he painted. And painted. And painted. Soon his little studio was very crowded. Navigating around stacks of abstract canvasses inhibited Howard's aggressive artistic style. To make room, Howard gave some of his paintings away; the rest he kept, as a reminder of what the mind can achieve in an idle moment.

With the demise of Tridont came a gleaming palette of opportunities waiting for the dip of Howard's entrepreneurial brush. Howard was ready to begin again, with a brand new company and a brand new plan. He paired up with a colleague he'd met way back in his Tridont days. His partner was in marketing, and Howard had more than a few products to market. He'd developed a line of tooth whiteners—toothpastes, mouthwashes, rinses—and was ready once again to invade the mouths of his fellow Canadians.

Canadians obliged by opening wide. The product was WhiteStep, and profits rose as people started adding it to their dental regimens. Which made Howard even busier. He'd already developed a brand new alcohol-free tooth whitener that worked, pushed hard and gotten it on the shelves, and managed to convince the public yet again that Dr. Howard knew best. Along the way he'd hobnobbed with beautiful famous people such as Heather Locklear and Christie Brinkley, who were chosen to help market the product based on the fine dental hygiene they exhibited. Lots of money, babes with nice teeth, and another product that worked, worked, worked. Howard was in his forties and in his element, on his third successful career with no sign of slowing.

Slow wasn't a word to describe Howard or his life. So

what was wrong with being in a hurry? He was a guy who knew where he was going and how he wanted to get there, and he lost no time doing just that. He was a businessman, he had things to do, he did them, they got done, he did some more. Why waste a minute? So much could be done on the road between point A and point B if you had a cellphone at your ear. God, he loved his cellphone. Whoever invented that thing was a genius! It meant never having to wait, and Howard hated to wait. Waiting meant being idle and that just wasn't in his nature. Even when he was relaxing, Howard always had to do something. Smash a tennis ball, hurl a football, zip around on a jet ski, jog a few miles on the treadmill. It was what being fit and active and successful and in the prime of your life was all about. Howard thought he had it down pat.

Who could ask for more out of life? Sometimes Howard would look around, amazed at what he'd managed to build, amazed at the family he'd built it for. His daughters had become young women and his wife was still a young woman. Together they'd gone through two decades, three homes, and far more ups than downs, thank God. Sometimes Howard would have to remind himself how lucky he really was. No matter how consumed he became with business, his family was his number-one priority.

But business ran a close second, and Howard poured his energy into putting his entrepreneurial vision into action. Canada was one market, but it certainly wasn't the only one, for a few miles south lay a nation of teeth just waiting to be whitened. But Howard had learned the hard way that expansion required money, and he wasn't keen to repeat the Tridont lesson.

Fortunately, he didn't have to—he'd learned enough the first time around to know he needed a partner with the business savvy to match his all-encompassing entrepreneurial style.

And he found that person quite by accident on a mild autumn day in 1993. Though it was a lazy Sunday morning for most, Howard had snapped on his rollerblades early in order to enjoy the combination of sunny skies and empty streets. Gliding through his neighborhood, he ran into Marty Teplitsky, his former legal counsel, equipped with bicycle and bagels. Then two things happened. Howard mentioned that he was trying to raise money for OraLife, his brand new venture. And Marty mentioned that his wife just happened to be good at that sort of thing.

Howard had never met Jennifer Jackson, but now he figured he ought to. So he followed Marty to convene an impromptu business meeting. It was 9 am Sunday morning. Who knew what could happen?

Jennifer Jackson was in her kitchen pouring a cup of coffee, enjoying a few minutes of relaxation on this Sunday morning. Jennifer was in her robe and pressed for time—she had a lot to do before catching a flight to Arizona later that day. She heard Marty come in. Good—fresh bagels. She turned around, expecting to be greeted by a poppy seed or two. Instead a stranger wearing black spandex zoomed into her kitchen on rollerblades.

Between the prospect of meeting a promising contact and the exhilaration of his early-morning blade, Howard was excited. He skidded to a halt in front of Jennifer, pumped her hand energetically and burst into an enthusiastic description of his current project. Marty remained in the background as he unpacked the bagels—he hadn't quite forgotten what his former client was like under the influence of adrenaline. Jennifer, who now needed her coffee even more, stood there in her robe and politely listened to the spandex-clad stranger in her kitchen.

Jennifer took another look at the gesticulating whirlwind in front of her. Who was this guy, exploding into her home unannounced to talk shop? She'd heard about Howard Rocket and Tridont, and was skeptical. But this guy wasn't what she'd expected. This was no flashy wheeler-dealer out for the quick buck. This was a person who was slowly drawing her in with his tremendous energy, who was winning her over with his raw enthusiasm, who was making her forget that she was in her robe and he was in form-fitting rollerblade garb on this very early Sunday morning, in the middle of her kitchen.

Jennifer agreed to continue the meeting later, under more traditional circumstances, but between now and then there was coffee to drink, a bagel to eat, and a flight to catch. As Howard rolled cheerfully out the door, she realized that she was already intrigued: beyond the casual exterior, Jennifer sensed in Howard Rocket the relentless pursuit of what he wanted. But that was okay, not only because she was equally intense but because she was interested. Very interested. They met, discussed, planned, strategized and agreed, forming an association that would successfully bear the fruits of finance and friendship over the next few years.

With Jennifer on board Howard's project started moving, smoothly progressing according to plan. They made an effective team. Things were getting done, and getting done efficiently. The best part was that Howard didn't have to worry about the details. Details were Jen's specialty. As usual, things were going great and Howard looked to the future with vigor and excitement. As usual, it didn't take long for the future to arrive.

During his operation of OraLife, a product called Chlorzoin had been invented at the University of Toronto. The product was a breakthrough in dentistry, because it far exceeded the scope of current preventive dental hygiene. When applied to the teeth, Chlorzoin attacked the *streptococci mutans* bacteria, largely responsible for tooth decay, thus preventing the formation of most cavities. The product had been proven, patented, and the rights to its production sold to Apotex, the largest generic drug manufacturer in Canada.

Apotex had the product, but it also had a problem: selling it. Chlorzoin could not be sold to pharmacies or over the counter because it had to be professionally applied. It couldn't be added to toothpaste or mouthwash, so it couldn't be marketed directly to the general public. Chlorzoin had to target the dental market. So Apotex decided that for specialized marketing it needed a specialist. And the name that kept coming up was Dr. Howard Rocket.

Howard was contacted by Apotex. They had heard about the product, and Howard decided that he wouldn't mind shaking up the dental profession one more time. Chlorzoin was a winner, but, more important it was a product that would dramatically improve the dental care received by the public, and ultimately reduce costs as well. But he wanted to make the project his own. Together with his contact at Apotex, he bought the rights to Chlorzoin and formed Knowell Therapeutic Technologies, Inc.—a company geared towards knowledge and wellness. And success would be okay, too.

Howard left the technical aspects of the pharmaceutical industry to his partner, instead applying his dental expertise to marketing strategies and his business expertise to obtaining the funds necessary for the company to prosper. Once again, that was where Jennifer came in. The combination of his vision and her meticulous and thorough style greatly reduced the risk of their joint ventures and established a fairly predictable recipe for success. Most important, working with Howard was fun. He loved his work, and exuded such positive energy that it was impossible to remain aloof. Jennifer found herself becoming excited about the possibilities of Chlorzoin, and joined Howard in raising the capital needed to fuel the successful operation of

Knowell. Their intention was to take the company public—and this time there would be no hard lessons to learn.

Howard was at the pinnacle of his life. Business was fantastic—exciting, creative, fast-paced, challenging and stimulating. He had the perfect life. How did he get so lucky? His family brought him such joy, his work was a pleasure, he had no financial clouds looming over his head. He had friends and hobbies and choices and freedom. He was fit and active and motivated and successful. He was liked by those who mattered and loved by those who really mattered. The present was bright. The future looked brighter.

Such was the state of Howard Rocket's life when he went to a pick-up football game in September 1995.

Stricken

Howard had always enjoyed sports. His tennis-playing days had never ended, and football, baseball, running, working out and generally staying fit had always been a non-negotiable part of his schedule. He was forty-seven years old and he looked damn good. Felt even better. And he planned to stay that way. So when his buddy Murray Belzberg called him up and invited him to a casual football game, he could think of no better way to spend a Sunday afternoon in mid-September. Murray had been playing football for twenty years, and assured Howard that this group would pose an agreeable athletic challenge.

Howard pulled on his running shoes. He really should be wearing cleats—who knew what state the ground would be in? But he'd gone shopping with Dana a while back and hadn't found shoes that he liked. Not that he was usually so picky, but none really interested him and he hadn't gotten around to finding ones that did. So plain runners would have to do, at least until he made it over to Sporting Life again.

Murray had been right—these guys played a good game of football. Howard was enjoying himself tremendously, keeping pace easily with players a decade or two younger than him. He got such a charge out of sports, out of the teamwork and the energy and the thrill. He zipped nimbly around the field, covering players, intercepting passes, and enjoying the freedom of an ordinary fall Sunday. He ran into position, and was open for a pass from the quarterback. The ball was coming right to him, and he was running to meet it. Intuitively, he knew it was high, so he jumped.

His hands met tough, weathered pigskin—and then his running shoes met sodden, trodden earth. No cleats. No grip. Howard's feet skidded out from under and his body lurched back beyond his control. His bottom hit first but his head kept going, smashing into the ground with a thud.

Howard opened his eyes and saw the worried faces of his teammates hovering over him. He was flat on his back and had been unconscious for about ten seconds. Gingerly, he sat up. His head throbbed a little, but he felt okay. He was ready to play some more. But his teammates were not in agreement, and parked him firmly under a tree to recuperate over a glass of water. Howard submitted at first, but watching others play made him restless. Hey, it was only a bump. He stretched a bit and walked it out. He felt fine. So he rejoined the game in the more relaxed position of steamboat-counter, and kept going until the group broke for the day.

He'd almost forgotten about the incident, really, until Murray called him a few days later to see how he was doing. And he was fine, he just had a bit of a headache, nothing a Tylenol couldn't handle. Howard was extremely busy, and his mind was on other things. Things with OraLife were moving quickly, it was all coming together, and required his full attention. He was going to Europe on business in a few days, he had a lot to do and it would be nice if this damn headache would go away.

Nice, but not necessary. Howard had too much to do, and he only really noticed the pain when he thought about it. It wasn't very distracting, just a dull ache behind his eyes. Howard went to Europe, came back, took meetings, worked out, led his life. Things were going well, as planned. Jen and he had been working around the clock on this thing, maybe that's why she had found him irritable at times. She was worried about him, said she didn't like the headaches. Well, he didn't like the headaches too much himself, but they weren't going to kill him. He made a mental note to see a doctor at some point in the future. Besides, most of the time he was himself. The occasional bad mood wasn't the end of the world.

Howard was in great shape, a month shy of forty-eight and looking at least ten years younger. He couldn't help it, he was proud of how fit he was and of the way he looked. But it did bother him that he was starting to get lines under his eyes; it made him look tired and God knows he was anything but that! He had thought about going in for some quick surgery to fix the problem, make him look more like how he felt. What the heck, he decided to go ahead with it. He scheduled the surgery for October 27, 1995. Dana would take him, he'd spend an hour, recuperate briefly, and look terrific. Friday October 27th—he looked forward to that day.

He just wished the damn headaches would go away. Most of the time his head felt okay, but sometimes the pain became fierce, searing momentarily across his brain and stopping him cold for a moment. Sometimes he couldn't quite see properly, things got a little blurry. Maybe it was just that he needed a stronger prescription. Maybe it was just that he was tired, he'd been working hard. Howard reminded himself to go see a doctor one of these days.

After all, he was forty-eight. He'd just advanced that much closer to the half-century mark the other day, a week before his operation. His family had had a party for him, with his sisters and their daughters and husbands. He chuckled to himself—all girls since him until Spencer, his niece Shawna's son. Judging from the family tree, it would be another forty or so years until the Rocket brood produced another boy. He didn't mind getting older as long as he didn't feel it, but why did everybody have to harp on it? He had no patience for that sort of thing. His sister, Marsha, had laughed and pointed out that he was getting on. Getting on? Where the hell was he going? He hadn't meant to snap at Marsha, but he had been annoyed.

Jennifer was really worried about him. Howard was not quite himself, and the combination of constant headaches, irritability and visual problems was troublesome. Why the hell was he going in for surgery under those circumstances? Who knew what complications could set in? But Howard was typically busy with life, and "what if's" weren't a huge priority. But she couldn't help being concerned. Howard would never make time to see a doctor. The symptoms were bad. He was a walking time bomb, primed for explosion at who knew what point?

Friday October 27th. Howard was home, resting until Dana drove him to Oakville for the operation that afternoon. The phone rang and he answered it, having no pressing reason to screen his calls. It was Jen, offering one last warning.

"Howard, something is wrong with you," she said with concern. Just as Howard was acting out of character, it was unusual for Jen to react this strongly. She was no alarmist, but right now she was pretty alarmed.

"Look, your symptoms are bad, really bad. They're classic indicators of stroke, Howard. Do you know what a stroke is like? It's like having a gun held to your head and then someone pulls the trigger. No second chances."

"Jen, I'm fine. Don't worry." What else could Howard say? He understood her concern but he didn't share it. No one else seemed to notice anything amiss. He appreciated it, but she was overreacting. In any case, he was going to see a doctor soon. He'd be fine. He felt fine. He was fine.

He heard the door open downstairs, heard the dogs go nuts. He checked his watch. Right on time. Dana had arrived to take him to the clinic and back before going for dinner at her boyfriend Michael's home. Howard, as always, looked forward to any time he got to spend with Dana, and the forty-minute drive to Oakville was infinitely improved by her presence.

After the long trip, the procedure seemed ridiculously short; Howard was in and out in barely half an hour. Having turned only a few pages in the waiting room Dana was called back to collect the patient. She followed the nurse to the recovery room and stopped suddenly, weak. Her father, her vibrant healthy father, lay pallid on a gurney, his eyes a swollen mess of deep, purple bruise. She felt faint. She had never seen her father seem so helpless. *Oh, my God*, she thought. *My God, I can't believe that's my father lying there.* The thought of her father ... she shuddered. She had to remind herself that he was fine, that it was just cosmetic eye surgery.

Dana drove her dad home, relieved to see her father back again. Howard fielded an anxious call from Debbie. Yes, he was fine, he was okay, he was going home to lie down, he'd see her there. And he was fine. He just wanted to lie down. Which he did as soon as he arrived home. Yes, he was okay. No, Dana didn't have to stay with him. She should go to Michael's for dinner, he'd be fine. Yes, he'd be okay for Debbie to go out and get him some medication. Painkillers, please. A lot. Yes, he was fine. Really. He just wanted to rest. Please.

Debbie and Dana left, and the house was quiet. God, he felt awful. He wished Debbie would come home with those painkillers. His head ... his eyes ... he didn't feel so good. Lie still. Sleep. But sleep wouldn't come and the pain was getting worse. His head was throbbing loudly, the pain was right up against his eyes, and oh, God, it hurt, it hurt. He felt his leg start to move up and down, and the pain deepened. He closed his eyes and willed his body to lie still but his body wouldn't listen. It wouldn't listen and the pain kept coming and his body kept shaking and oh God it hurt so much. Using the last bit of energy his body could muster, Howard flung his arm toward the phone, his flailing fingers finding the numbers 9-1-1 and pressing, his head pounding, his mouth dry. *Please come soon please come soon please come soon* he thought as his body shook and his head throbbed and the pain grew still deeper. The phone rang shrilly, exploding in his skull. It was Debbie on the cellphone. She wanted to know if he wanted some ice cream. Howard said thickly in a voice that sounded strange: "I'm not feeling so good. Come home." *Come home please come home.*

Debbie felt her body go cold. She had been driving north, but before she knew it she had done a u-turn and was zooming home, her heart racing. *Oh my God, I never should have left him.* She veered wildly into her driveway and leapt out of the car and up the stairs to her husband. His color was gray, his body was wracked with spasm. His head hurt, his head hurt. She called 911 again, *hurry, please hurry*. And they did, because suddenly they were there and the dogs were going crazy. A woman and a man, asking questions, and she said, *my husband is having a stroke,* and the woman said to Howard, *let me grab your hands* and his body still had feeling and movement, and they put Howard in a wheelchair to get him down the stairs while the dogs whipped around their legs in a frenzy, and Debbie had to leave Howard for a moment to put them away.

He felt himself being carried unevenly down the stairs, and the pain was still there and he felt nausea welling up inside him and pushing its way out. The ambulance attendant warned his partner, *don't leave him by himself* and Howard felt the nausea push higher and he asked for a bag and he got one and the nausea pushed more and burst out of him and he was sick. And he felt himself being put into the back of the ambulance in slow motion, and then he was looking down on himself, looking at himself colored gray and clutching another plastic bag just in case, and he saw the other attendant on his left giving him oxygen and he heard them tell the driver to go to the Mount Sinai Hospital and then he didn't see or hear any more.

A Twelve-Hour Window

There was no real reason for Dana Rocket to call home. She'd just left, for God's sake. It was Friday night and she had nothing else to do but enjoy a leisurely meal with her boyfriend's family. She'd call after dinner; her dad was probably resting.

And yet. And yet Dana felt like calling—more than that, she needed to call. Maybe the sight of her dad all ashen and bruised had shaken her up, maybe she was giving in to an irrational fear she never knew she had. Whatever the reason, she wanted to make contact, just to be sure everything was okay. She and her dad spoke on the phone all the time. She certainly didn't need a *reason* to call him. She'd call, say hi, then relax and enjoy her dinner.

Michael Kalles was upstairs when he heard his sister calling him frantically back down again. He raced downstairs. He heard Dana's sobs before he saw her clutching the phone in the kitchen, her face red and blotchy from crying and looking suddenly old, so very, very old. He felt a small stab of fear.

"My dad—my dad's in the hospital." Dana struggled to get out the words between sobs. "He—I don't know, my mom said—he called the ambulance himself—and he was alone, he was all *alone*!" She was hyperventilating and very quickly losing control. Michael felt another stab. Strong, he had to be strong for Dana. Hell, he needed strength himself—Howard was like a second father to him. Putting his arms around Dana, Michael gently took the phone away and spoke to Debbie himself.

"Debbie, what's going on? Is he all right?" Michael couldn't conceive of any other possibility.

Debbie's voice was heavy. "It doesn't look good."

Michael hadn't known he was holding his breath until he exhaled heavily. "We're on our way."

Less than a minute later they were out of the driveway and on the way to the hospital. Dana was a mess. All the vague, horrible fears of this afternoon were back with a vengeance, crowding her mind with possibilities too frightening to consider.

"Dana, Dana, he's going to be okay, he is, of course he is." Michael was trying to comfort her, but he believed his words. It was a probably side effect of the surgery. It happens all the time. The hospitals know how to handle it. But Dana wouldn't, couldn't be comforted. Her whole world was crumbling as her best friend, her father, lay sick in some hospital bed—and where the hell was she? She never should have left him. Oh God, what was taking them so long? When they reached the hospital, Michael was about to park but Dana was already flying out the door and into the emergency room where she needed to see her father, now.

And there he was. *Oh my God, what was wrong with him?* His skin was gray beneath the oxygen mask covering his face, and his left side was jerking spasmodically. The pain on his face made her wince. She rushed to him, crying harder than before. He looked at her, and through his pain she saw in his face that he knew she was there, and that he was glad, and she was glad, too, because he was alert, but more than that he was *alive*. Dana was overwhelmed by love for her dad and she poured it out to him, trying to infuse him with life through her presence.

Howard was aware of everything from somewhere behind the pain. He had thrown up all the way to the hospital, his gut churning angrily in time with the pounding of his head. He couldn't get his left side to stop shaking, his leg was moving up and down violently and he had no control. And his head still hurt so much.

"They don't know what it is, it may just be a very severe migraine." Dana hadn't even noticed her mother, sitting quietly beside the bed. She hadn't seen anything but her father. Debbie gave Dana and Michael the rundown as Howard's leg thrashed about on the bed. Howard could not speak; when he got to the hospital they had put a tube in his mouth. He had tried to scream and get them to take it out but he couldn't unclench his teeth. Now he joined the conversation with his eyes as his daughter's sweaty hand gripped his own.

"But if it's not a migraine..." Dana needed to know everything. She looked at her mother, who looked so tired, and so worried, and so scared. There was something else.

Debbie wanted to be reassuring, but it was difficult. "If it's not a migraine, I don't know, they just can't tell at this point. But"—Debbie's voice caught—"it could be a stroke."

Howard didn't want them to worry. He would be okay, he was in pain but he wasn't afraid. Debbie was with him and they were in the hospital, which was more than half the battle. He wasn't afraid. He tried to tell Dana and Michael that, but the words couldn't come and his teeth wouldn't release. He'd be fine. Here, he had Raptors tickets. He wouldn't be using them, that much he knew. They should take them and get out of the damn hospital on a Friday night.

He locked on Dana and Michael with his eyes, and tried to tell them.

Dana was leaning over him, there with him, for him. "Dad, what is it?" Her voice trembled. God, she was so scared. "We're here, Daddy, we're here." Michael moved closer, into his field of vision. Howard tried to show them. He lifted his arm and slam-dunked a few times.

Panic was rising in Dana. Oh, God, what was he trying to say? Now Howard was pointing at them, at her and Michael. He was scaring her. His arm moved more wildly as her dad tried urgently to communicate, pointing at Dana, then Michael, then back again.

Michael rushed to Dana's side and put his hand over Howard's. "I love your daughter, I'll take care of her, I promise." The words tumbled out of Michael as Dana turned to stare, in shock, first at her boyfriend and then at her father. Howard's gesticulations became more frantic. He shook his head and slam-dunked more furiously. Dana was sobbing again.

"Don't worry, Daddy, don't worry," said Dana. "We're all going to be okay, it's going to be okay." And Michael: "I promise, I'll take care of your daughter."

Howard shook his head again, and held up his hand in frustration. Stop. Dana and Michael fell silent, confused. Once more, he tried to show them. Slowly, slowly, so they could get it. With effort, Howard lifted his hand and dribbled the ball. Then he stopped, lifted the ball in an arc, and sent it spinning into the basket, following its descent with his eyes. Three points.

He looked at them, exhausted. *Now* did they get it?

It took them a second, but they got it. And in the midst of the fear and the worry, they laughed. Basketball. *Basketball!* They laughed harder. Michael was practically proposing and he wanted them to catch a Raptors game! Dana wasn't sure where her tears were coming from anymore, she didn't know how she could squeeze a laugh out of this horrifying nightmare, but there they were, four people living and laughing under the pale yellow pulse of the fluorescent lights.

Howard was laughing with them. See? He'd be okay.

But his leg wouldn't stop moving.

The laughter faded. Dana took her father's hand again, and Debbie took his other hand, and together they sat, waiting, until someone came to tell them what was going on.

◆ ◆ ◆

The phone rang a few times, and then the answering machine picked up. In Tokyo, Amie Rocket left a message for her dad to call her.

◆ ◆ ◆

Dr. Metra, the resident who had admitted Howard to the Mount Sinai Hospital, now returned with Dr. Shandling, the neurologist on duty. As Debbie, Dana and Michael looked on anxiously, Dr. Shandling expertly tested Howard's body for reflexes. Right foot, okay. Left foot. Nothing. She repeated the test. Left foot. Nothing. Then she probed up Howard's left side.

"Can you feel this?" Howard shook his head. She moved higher. "This?" Again, no. She moved to his right side. Howard nodded. He could feel that.

Dr. Shandling turned to face them. "The loss of feeling and motor control on one side indicates a stroke," she explained. "Although it could still be a migraine, the jagged vision and the throwing up are all typical of strokes. I think you should be prepared." She turned to Howard. "Dr. Rocket, we've contacted Dr. Lozano at the Western Division of the Toronto Hospital, which is one of the best neurological centers in North America. He's arranging your transfer and assembling a team over there. If this is a stroke, we have to move fast because right now something's blocking the passage of blood to your brain, and we need to unclog the blockage in time or else there will be permanent damage. We're looking at a twelve-hour window, at most. Do you understand all this?" Howard nodded. The twelfth hour since his stroke was nearing.

It seemed Debbie couldn't breathe. Twelve hours? How did they know? How long had they already been there? It felt like a year, a lifetime, since she'd gone out to pick up a prescription. If they had so little time, *what the hell were they waiting for?*

Dr. Shandling went on. "If it is a stroke, we don't have many options. We could inject you with an anti-coagulant, which is a blood-thinning agent. But there's no guarantee that thinning your blood will reduce the clot significantly, or even at all."

"What will?" Michael asked. He didn't want to hear about what wasn't going to help Howard. There was no time for that.

"There is an experimental procedure that, if it works, will attack the clot directly and break it up so that circulation is re-established."

Debbie was alarmed. "Experimental?"

"It's been used on heart attacks for some time now, but only recently on strokes," Dr. Shandling said. "A dye is injected into the bloodstream, which travels through the circulatory system. The interruption of the flow of dye indicates that the blood vessel in the brain is obstructed either by a narrowing or by a clot. If the angiographic picture suggests a clot, then the interventional neuroradiologist injects a substance that essentially 'blasts' the clot, dissolving and fragmenting it into small pieces so that the artery unclogs. We know that it works, but the risks are high."

"What are the risks?" Dana asked.

"Well," Dr. Shandling began, "there's the risk that little pieces of the original clot can lodge elsewhere in the brain, causing other, smaller strokes. Where a stroke occurs in the brain determines what functions are impaired, so further damage is likely, if that happens." Dr. Shandling turned to Howard. "Okay so far?" Howard nodded, more weakly this time. She went on.

"But you have to weigh the risks not only against the other alternatives, but also in light of the patient. Dr. Rocket is in otherwise excellent physical shape, and he's still a young man. He's conscious and alert, and seems to have sustained no further damage since the original stroke. His chances with this procedure are better than most."

"Better than most!" Debbie couldn't believe what she was hearing. "Isn't there anything else that can be done?"

Dr. Shandling shook her head. "Not with strokes. The brain can't function without fresh oxygenated blood. If this goes untreated, then ultimately there will be brain damage. At least." She turned to Howard. "Dr. Rocket, crucial hours have already elapsed since your stroke. This decision has to be made, and made now. As your doctor, I'm advising you to undergo the procedure, but it's your decision. Do you understand all I've just said?" Howard nodded. It wasn't the greatest news he'd ever had but the doctors knew what they were doing, and he wasn't in much of a position to choose.

"Dr. Rocket, you can either die, be permanently disabled, or undergo this procedure."

There really wasn't much of a choice.

Ripples

They spent most of the night at the Sinai, waiting for the go-ahead from the Western to bring Howard over. They'd moved him from the ER to a room by the intensive care unit where he could be monitored. Howard had finally succeeded in sending Dana and Michael home, but Debbie hadn't left his side. She sat with him as the hours inched past, waiting, waiting, as the twelve-hour window narrowed inexorably and tomorrow became today.

The sky was still dark when they came for him.

5:05 AM
It had been over ten hours since his stroke and there was no time to lose. Howard was still conscious, but barely. His left side had stopped its jerking and now his whole body was still. The tube in his mouth had been removed, at least, but words came with great difficulty and exhausting effort. Only his eyes were alert as he was wheeled urgently along the hall to the angiosuite where his clot would be unmasked and targeted. Debbie hurried to keep up with her husband as they slammed open doors and swung around corners. She'd been up all night but didn't notice, didn't care.

She caught a glimpse of a big man in surgical greens, and then the doors to the angiography swung shut behind her husband. The wait had begun.

6:08 AM

Dr. Hu worked quickly; he knew it had been over ten hours since the patient's stroke. He'd have to obtain images of Howard's brain vessels to locate the obstruction before anything could be done. Deftly, he made an incision near Howard's groin and inserted a catheter into his vertebral artery, carefully following it up to the base of his brain. He injected the dye that would confirm the location of the clot for blasting. It would take ten or twelve seconds for the dye to set before the x-ray. Dr. Hu glanced at his patient. He seemed out of it. It was clear that he was very ill, and yet ... it was also clear that he was there, somehow. Something in his eyes, he seemed to blink knowingly at you. This guy wanted to live.

Ten seconds, eleven, twelve. Dr. Hu snapped the shot. Now they could get to work.

6:09 AM

Howard was used to the pain now, he almost didn't notice it as he drifted in and out of awareness. He had no idea how long it had been since his head had exploded upstairs in his bedroom, had no idea of time, didn't notice it passing.

New pain hit him hard. The blunted throb of his head was momentarily silenced by the pain emanating from his groin. He felt something spreading slowly within him, felt it moving in his limbs, seeping through him. *Hurts, hurts.* He tried to tell them but he couldn't talk and he couldn't move. He couldn't do anything but let the pain wash over him and welcome the drift as it drew him back down into darkness.

6:12 AM

Debbie sat nervously in the waiting area. The situation was out of her hands. She had called their friend, Kenny Field, and got the name of the best neurosurgeon available. He was on his way. Now it was up to Howard.

6:15 AM

The darkness veiling Howard's eyes started to shimmer as little pinpricks of light shone through. His head still hurt, and he still felt the pain from the catheter. He was conscious of being flat on his back, and he heard the voice above him telling him to hold still, not to move, they were going to take a picture. He wasn't sure if the light behind was from the picture, or if it was part of his stroke, but it grew stronger as the dye filled his body. Three of the pinpricks swelled and grew, swimming in front of his eyes in shades of black and gold. He thought they were neurons but he wasn't sure. They moved back and forth in concert with the little pinpricks, melting through the darkness and filling his head with light. Then, slowly, the image faded and the darkness crept in once more.

6:23 AM

Dr. Hu was examining the x-ray when Dr. Willinsky, the interventional neuroradiologist, arrived. He studied the charts.

"Left hemiplegia. How's his right side?" asked Dr. Willinsky.

"Seems fine, he can move," replied Dr. Hu. "And he was awake, functioning mentally according to his wife. There hasn't been further deterioration since the initial attack." Dr. Hu indicated the x-ray, pointing out a dark patch at the base of the brain. "Occlusion in the basilar artery."

Basilar thrombosis. Rare. Dr. Willinsky would see a basilar stroke (posterior circulation) for every hundred or so frontal strokes (anterior circulation) he saw. There was a lot that wasn't yet known about these strokes, but Dr. Willinsky did know that their window for successful treatment was generally wider. For other areas of the brain, after four to six hours, forget it. But with the basilar artery, the sudden blockage in blood supply was offset by collateral flow from different areas, which gave the patient some extra time. But this one was already in the tenth hour, there wasn't a whole lot of time left. Left untreated, basilar strokes were lethal.

Options: inject anti-coagulant or blast the clot with urokinase. Dr. Willinsky knew that his patient was a very sick man, and that the option of merely thinning his blood didn't offer much hope. There was a lot to salvage in this patient: conscious, good mental capacity, excellent physical condition. Present neurological evidence favored aggressive treatment. If they eliminated the clot, blood flow would be re-established and further damage prevented. But if they didn't ...

No buts. They'd give the clot-blasting a shot. It was, he suspected, the patient's only hope.

6:25 AM

Debbie tried to sleep, God knows she was tired enough, she should be out like a light. But sleep eluded her; her exhaustion couldn't compete with her fear. Every so often her eyes would stray to the clock on the wall, and she would be amazed at how slowly the minute hand was moving. Time seemed to be stretched out in this never-ending night.

Suddenly, there were Dana and Michael, running down the hallway to her.

"Mom, Mom, is he all right?" Dana wished she hadn't left. What if something had happened?

"He's in there with them now." She touched Dana's hand. "Honey, he'll be okay. The odds are with him and he's a fighter. When have you known your father to quit?"

The words comforted Dana. Her mom was right. Her father wouldn't quit.

She sighed. It was time to let the rest of the family in on this nightmare. She walked over to the payphone and dropped in her first quarter.

6:27 AM

The first catheter was still in place, a path up the patient's vertebral artery to the base of his brain. Dr. Willinsky inserted a second, smaller catheter into the first and threaded it carefully up toward the blockage. Inside the inner catheter was a guidewire, which allowed the doctor to control the paths taken through the multitude of tiny passages bringing fresh blood to the brain. He nodded to Dr. Hu, who snapped a picture. In a few moments they studied it, gauging their distance from the clot. Dr. Willinsky carefully rotated the wire for direction, coaxing the catheter along another passage. Dr. Hu snapped a second picture. It was this tedious process of looking and guiding that would eventually bring them to the clot. Tedious, but life-saving.

6:40 AM

Kelli Young was disoriented. Strange bed, no landmarks, total darkness and why was she awake? Another insistent ring of the telephone gave her the answer. She groped beside her, feeling for where her sister Shawna kept her phone. Where was it? As she twisted toward the ringing, she caught the dim red glow of the alarm clock. She groaned. 6:40. Reaching for the phone, she cursed herself for agreeing to stay with Shawna and Steven's kids while they were away for the weekend. The phone kept ringing. God, it was so loud. She fumbled for a few seconds and managed to find the receiver in the darkness. She mumbled a thick hello.

"Kelli? Kelli?" The voice was shrill and panicked and woke her up in a hurry.

"Jill? Is that you? What's going on?" Why was her sister calling this early?

Jill was crying as she told her. "It's Uncle Howie, he's sick, Kel, he had a stroke. He's in the hospital. That's where I am right now."

Kelli was stunned. Her uncle was such a healthy guy, it couldn't be possible. Her mom, Tyrral, was in Florida. "Jill, did you call Mom and Dad?"

"Not yet."

"And Shawna and Steven, and Missy, and Marsha ... okay, you get in touch with Mom and Dad and I'll call Shawna and Steven. You call Missy. I'll be right over."

7:00 AM

Nothing beat Florida. They had been there a week and Tyrral and Sonny Prashker were by no means ready to come home. A good thing, too, because they had a few more weeks in Florida and then a cruise to look forward to. There were definitely perks to having grown-ups for kids.

But right now one of those grown-ups was sobbing on the other end of the telephone as her mother tried desperately to wake up and figure out what the hell was going on. Tyrral was grimly aware that at seven in the morning, it couldn't be good.

Jill was crying. She was at the hospital, Uncle Howard had a blood clot, she didn't know where, she didn't know anything but that he'd collapsed and been rushed to the hospital, and he couldn't move, and she had to come home right away.

Tyrral struggled to remain calm. "Jill, is Debbie there? Put her on." A beat, and then Debbie was on the line.

"Debbie, my God, what's wrong with him?"

Debbie was composed, surprisingly so. "Tyrral, last night Howard had a stroke. So far, that's all they can tell us."

Tyrral groped beside her for Sonny's hand, as though that would help. "Is he going to be okay?"

Debbie was still composed, but barely. "Well," she said, "it's life-threatening."

The words fell like a blow on Tyrral's brain. This just couldn't be happening. Howie was such a healthy guy, she'd just seen him, he looked great. But Debbie hadn't needed to say any more. Tyrral felt everything falling in on her, and strained to keep her mind clear. Tickets. They needed to change their tickets, to pack and check out and get on the first plane back to Toronto. She turned to Sonny beside her, but he was already up and hurling their stuff into suitcases. He moved quickly and efficiently, but his hands were shaking. Howard, oh, my God ...

No time to lose. She grabbed the phone and hit zero.

7:15 AM
Marsha Baker had gotten a late start this Saturday morning; usually she was already out running. Better get going, it was almost November, there wouldn't be too many more Saturday mornings like this. She was pulling on her Reeboks when the phone rang. Who was calling this early? She picked up the phone.

"Auntie Marsha, it's Missy." Her niece wasn't normally in the habit of early-morning phone calls. Marsha felt her stomach tighten. What was going on?

"Missy, my God, is everything all right?"

"It's Uncle Howie, he's in the hospital, he's got a brain tumor or something, I don't know." Marsha's stomach clenched some more. "Dana just called me from the hospital. Right now he's still awake, that's a good sign. Dana said Uncle Howie wants us to bring Bubby to the hospital."

An involuntary smile. Trust Howard to organize things from a hospital bed. Then the smile faded. What was Howard doing in a hospital bed? She had to see him.

"Stay put, Missy, I'll be right over."

7:25 AM

It was almost 1:30 in the afternoon, Tokyo time. Amie left another message for her parents and hung up the phone.

7:40 AM

They were near now, had almost reached the clot, at which point the real work would begin. The most recent angiogram confirmed that they were down to the last minutes of probing and guiding within the patient's cranial circulatory system. Dr. Hu began preparing the injection of urokinase, the substance that would break up the clot under the onslaught of its chemical stream—if they were lucky.

Dr. Willinsky glanced at the clock. They were still within the twelve-hour window, but barely. Time to narrow the gap. With another rotation of the guidewire, the catheter slipped further along inside Howard's brain.

8:00 AM

Risa Rocket was asleep. Deeply, wonderfully asleep. Thank God, she needed to sleep, to recharge, to get away. Hence this weekend getaway with her new husband to a little cottage in Bracebridge. And since their arrival her body had been emptied of tension and sleep had come easily and soundly, and it felt so good to sleep, and that's why she had ignored the phone and that's why she was ignoring Eddie who was shaking her, reaching into her slumber and pulling her reluctantly toward another morning. She clung to her sleep, willing the outside world away. She tried not to hear Eddie's voice drifting toward her through a haze.

"Risa, Risa, you're brother isn't well."

The haze vanished. Her husband was no alarmist, but there was something heavy in his voice that yanked her awake. Howard. Howard. Oh, God. She sat up and reached for the phone.

8:05 AM

The phone rang. Shawna Page had been fast asleep, but this was her first time leaving her kids and some internal mechanism was attuned to that fact. She and her husband Steven were celebrating their fifth wedding anniversary in New York City—alone. It had been a step that she'd taken resolutely, if a bit nervously. And so, with the first ring she was alert, her mind already at home with Spencer and Sydney, the first stirrings of apprehension taking shape in her chest. *It's probably some sick practical joke, wishing us an early happy anniversary*, she thought ruefully. *Anniversary wishes at 8 in the morning I don't need.* But her thoughts were on her kids as she picked up the phone.

By the time she replaced the receiver she and Steven were both crying, anniversary plans forgotten, driven only by the need to be at Howie's side. Her uncle was a role model to both of them, the godfather to their son, the robust picture of success and joy and life. She couldn't reconcile that image with the chilling description her sister had just given.

But she would have to, and the sooner the better. Right now she and Steven had to get moving and get the hell out of New York. Between the two of them, they were packed, checked out and in a cab to La Guardia at 8:25. Happy anniversary.

By nine o'clock they were on the plane.

Straight Answers

They were there. The angiogram showed that the catheter tip was inside the clot, ready to attack it from the inside out. Dr. Willinsky and Dr. Hu exchanged a glance. What they were about to do was risky, because it could trigger another stroke. They doubted that their patient could live through that. But there were no doubts about his chances with this stroke: he had none if they didn't do something, fast. And it had to be fast, because their twelve hours were waning and his brain had been without blood for too long already. Tissue was dying. They had to move.

Dr. Willinsky placed the tip of the hypodermic needle into the inner catheter and carefully depressed the plunger. Urokinase began to seep into the catheter. He felt the resistance of the liquid as it was forced out of the needle, felt his answering pressure propel it forward. It was making a beeline for the clot, which would disintegrate and dissolve under the potency of its onslaught. They hoped.

Dr. Hu did another angiogram. Together they studied the picture. The clot was definitely smaller, but not by much. They'd have to keep injecting until it was gone. In the meantime, the catheter had to be adjusted again. Dr. Willinsky rotated the wire, his eyes moving often to the x-ray to determine his direction. He turned to Dr. Hu, who already had the second injection prepared. In seconds the urokinase was speeding toward the clot for round two. Then three. Then four. Then five.

Howard lay motionless, dimly aware of the confrontation taking place in his brain. By now the new pain had blended with the old into a constant throb. He hovered near the threshold of consciousness, drifting in and out. He knew that the doctors were there because he could hear their voices through the dense fog surrounding his head.

"Almost there." Dr. Willinsky's voice was grimly satisfied. After more than ten hits of urokinase, the clot was at last near oblivion. Blood had finally begun to trickle past the blockage to nourish the parched brain of their patient. It was only a trickle, but it was constant.

It was Dr. Hu who noticed the dark spot deeper in the brain. "Another one, distal vessel." He pointed. "We'll have to go in and open it up."

Dr. Willinsky nodded. It was not unexpected for broken pieces of the clot to lodge elsewhere. "That one he can live with. We'll get to it after we've eradicated the main blockage." Dr. Hu nodded and passed him another urokinase injection.

And another.
And another.
And another.

Another worried visitor approached the nursing station asking about a Dr. Howard Rocket. The on-duty nurse no longer had to check on where this patient was located; by now, she definitely knew. She repeated what she'd told all the others and watched him hurry down the hall toward the waiting room, wondering who this Dr. Howard Rocket was to bring so many people to his side this early on a Saturday morning.

It was no longer early to Kenny Field, who'd been awakened by Debbie's frantic phone call at six AM. He'd made a call, had gotten the name of the best neurosurgeon at Toronto Western Hospital, and had called Debbie back. Then he made a few calls of his own, quietly letting people know what had happened to their friend.

Now he was at the hospital—again. He knew hospitals—knew their smell, their taste, their feel. He'd spent months in one, recuperating from a ski accident that had nearly paralyzed him, an event that lived on in the constantly throbbing left arm that would never quite heal. Now he felt the past engulf him as he approached the bewildered-looking cluster of people in the waiting room.

Debbie was there, at the center, under control and in control. Kenny found himself slightly surprised by this, and realized that he would have expected the sweet, somewhat reserved Debbie he knew to be the type to break down in confusion and helplessness. This woman was concerned, yet calm, keeping the emotions of those around her in check.

Kenny looked around at the family members. He knew most of them from his close association with the Rocket clan—Howard's sister Marsha with her husband Shelly; his mother, looking old and frightened; three of Tyrral's daughters; and Michael, Dana's boyfriend. And of course Dana, who was clearly overcome.

The calm projected by Debbie had obviously not reached her daughter, whose grief and fear were written all over her face. Kenny could see her focusing on Howard, willing him to get better, praying for it. He wondered where Amie was, if she knew. He thought about asking, decided against it, thought about it again, changed his mind. He knew how important it had been to him to have his kids there for him.

Amie. Debbie just didn't know. Tokyo was so far away, and Amie was so alone. How could she expect her daughter to hop on a plane with no comfort or support, isolated and out of touch for eighteen long, lonely, frightening hours? Who knew what she would be coming home to? Nobody said the word *funeral* but it was there, filling the room with unspoken implication. Is that what her daughter would come home to? She felt fear building inside her again, and she pushed it down. *Composure. Control.* Howie wasn't around to make the decisions anymore. She needed to keep her head clear.

God, she was weary. This night that had changed her life was never-ending. She wanted to shut her eyes against the world and open them again to the simplicity of yesterday. She wanted to cast off the weight of decisions to be made. She wanted the doctors to come out and tell her that everything was okay so that she could clean out her churning mind with a single, pure wave of relief. She could almost feel it.

"Mrs. Rocket?" She looked up. Two doctors were standing before the small crowd of family. Debbie recognized the younger one as the man she had seen earlier. The other one spoke.

"I'm Dr. Willinsky, your husband's neuroradiologist. We've just completed the procedure." You could hear a pin drop. He looked out at them. Fear, expectation, hope. This was the worst part of his job. "We were successful in eliminating the clot and re-establishing blood flow. Beyond that, we can't be sure. Dr. Rocket's basilar artery was blocked for a very long time. Enough time for significant damage to have been done to his brain. Right now he's alive and that's better than most, but he is a very, very sick man." He turned to his colleague. "Dr. Hu can answer any questions you may have."

Dr. Hu felt eleven pairs of eyes swivel and fasten onto him. He wished he could give them good news. But the next best thing was to give them straight answers; it was the least he could do for these people. He sat down gently before them, at eye-level.

"I'm Dr. Hu, the neuroradiology fellow on this case. Dr. Rocket had a blockage in his basilar artery, which is the main supply of blood to the brainstem. In order to unblock it, we inserted a catheter into his vertebral artery and injected dye into his bloodstream. This stained the clot so it would be visible on an x-ray." They were all looking at him, searching for a glimmer of hope. Dr. Hu wished he could give it to them.

"Once we knew the exact location of the clot, we inserted a smaller catheter into the first one and threaded it up toward Dr. Rocket's blocked basilar artery. Through this second catheter we applied a large quantity of a clot-busting enzyme called urokinase to the affected area. It works somewhat like a drain cleaner, unclogging the artery and letting the blood through." He looked at them, saw that they understood, and went on. "This procedure is not without risk. There is the danger that parts of the broken clot can trigger another stroke. This occurred in Dr. Rocket's case."

Dana felt anger building inside her. They were supposed to help her father, not make him worse! She looked at her mother. Debbie's eyes were closed, but only for a moment. She opened them and looked at the doctor, waiting for him to explain.

"We were able to remove the second clot after we had finished with the first one. The initial clot was by far the more dangerous. If that had not been eliminated, he would have died."

"And now?" Dana's voice was sharper than she'd meant, shrill and a little unsteady. Michael took her hand and squeezed it gently.

"Blood flow from the basilar artery was cut off for at least eleven hours. Fortunately, collateral flow from other areas allowed some blood to reach that region, but it would not have been nearly enough to offset the deprivation caused by the clot. It is very likely that Dr. Rocket sustained significant damage to the affected areas of the brain." He heard someone give a little moan.

Debbie needed something more concrete than this. What would this ultimately mean for Howie, for all of them? "What kind of damage?"

"Mrs. Rocket, that's something we can't know yet. Your husband has retained consciousness for the most part and exhibited signs of mental awareness. He's young and in excellent physical shape, and he's got the blood vessels of a twenty-year-old. But brain damage is irreversible, and his artery was blocked for a long, long time." Dr. Hu could see the last traces of hope ebbing out of Debbie's face, and he felt a sudden surge of sadness. Every day brought new tragedies in his line of work. She was still looking at him, and he realized that he hadn't answered her question. *How do you tell someone that life will never be the same, that her husband will probably be in a vegetative state, if he lives at all?* "Because so many bodily functions are controlled by the brain, it's impossible to say what will happen. The stroke could affect breathing, swallowing, speech, motor control, vision, mental capacity. All of these areas could be damaged, or just one of them. We won't be able to assess the extent of the damage until he regains a sufficient degree of consciousness."

"When...?" Dana asked, needing to know.

Kenny Field knew the doctor didn't have an answer. No one could tell where the body might go from here.

Dr. Hu sighed, and levelled with the people sitting before him. "Right now, Dr. Rocket has suffered an incredible trauma to his brain. He almost died. We're going to do all we can to keep him alive, but there can be no guarantees. The next twenty-four hours will be critical. We can only wait and see what unfolds."

Unfolds. Unravels was more like it—Dana's whole world was coming apart. *Significant damage ... irreversible ... incredible trauma ... no guarantees.* Dr. Hu was standing up. "They'll be moving him from the OR to Neuro Intensive Care very shortly." There was nothing more he could do for them right now. "I'm very sorry I wasn't able to bring you better news, but I hope I will be able to do so very soon. Please don't hesitate to ask if you have any questions. I will be available; have the nurses page me." He would have said something else, but he couldn't think of anything. But he'd be back.

Dana watched him go. She wouldn't ask if her father would live. She couldn't accept that as a question. But behind the medical caution the message had been unmistakable, coming from the man who moments ago had been in her father's brain. *Prepare for the worst. Expect nothing. No guarantees. No!* She refused to accept anything that undermined her hope. Her father's body had betrayed him, but he was still alive. With so much to live for, he would cling to that life with the will and the drive that was his trademark. Everything was still possible. Her dad would make it so.

She was suddenly aware of the people around her; she hadn't really noticed anyone else while Dr. Hu was speaking. Her grandmother was crying softly, and Dana went to her, kneeling in front of her and taking her hands. Helen was whimpering softly, repeating the words "My son, why my son?" like a mantra. She was so confused, it had all happened so fast. Marsha and Missy had picked her up and taken her to the hospital, but no one would tell her why. They said he had had an accident, he had hit his head, but that he was okay. Marsha

had mentioned something about elective surgery, nothing serious, they did it all the time. Helen had been worried but she
had believed them, believed that she would see her son walk
out of those big double doors with a bandage and a smile,
laughing at his old mother for overreacting. And now this doctor
was telling her that her son had had a stroke, that he might
never get up from his hospital bed, when it was just supposed
to be a little bump on his head. Helen felt weak. How could
she stand it? *I'll never live through this,* she thought.

"Yes you will, Bubby, and he will, too." Dana was there with
her, and Helen realized that she had spoken aloud. She covered
her granddaughter's hand with her own and sat, thinking.

The family sat together quietly, each absorbing what they
had been told. Kenny noticed Dr. Hu further down the hall
with a nurse and, on impulse, got up and walked toward him.
Kenny had been impressed with the way the young doctor had
handled the family; he'd waited for questions, used lay terms,
hadn't rushed. Kenny thought he ought to let him know that
someone had noticed. Dr. Hu turned to him expectantly as he
approached, signalling that he was willing to be interrupted.
True to his word, he thought.

"Dr. Hu. I'm Ken Field, a friend of the Rocket family. I
want to let you know that I was impressed with your sensitiv-
ity in handling the family. They need the kind of balance and
compassion you provided. Thank you."

Dr. Hu thanked him, pleased that he'd been able to do
something for the family, however small. But it wouldn't matter
much. He glanced down the hall toward the waiting room and
lowered his voice.

"Mr. Field," he said gravely, "I think you should get the
family ready. I doubt that he will live."

The Unbroken Circle

Now there was nothing to do but wait. Howard's family and friends sat there together, filling time with subdued conversation or simply with their own thoughts. Occasionally someone would use the phone. There was talk of practicalities; Howard's business associates would be notified, Missy would take the dogs for a few days, Marsha would look after calling some friends. Empty conversation filling up empty hours.

Word had spread, and as the day wore on the crowd in the waiting room grew larger. Shawna and Stephen had gone straight from the airport to the hospital, wearing matching expressions of pallor and fear. Jennifer Jackson had rushed over immediately, sickened and shocked that her prediction of Howard's stroke had come true. She couldn't help feeling guilty that she should have done more. Amie's boyfriend, Michael Wuls, was there with his family. He hadn't seen Amie's family much since she had left for Tokyo, but he had just taken Howard out for a birthday dinner the week before, and he had seemed fine, great, his old self. He found it hard to believe that this was happening. They were all still waiting for Tyrral and Sonny to arrive, and Risa, but they were coming, on their way, converging like the rest of them to this one little waiting room in the Western Division of Toronto Hospital.

Howard had since been transferred to the ICU, and they hadn't been allowed to visit yet. They'd seen him briefly though, once. Helen had seen him being wheeled down the hall, lying motionless on a hospital bed. It seemed to Helen that there were pipes and tubes going into every part of him, and his face ... she was too old for this, her heart couldn't take this kind of shock. Her son's face was a mass of purple swollen bruises over grayish, dead-looking skin. She remembered he'd had surgery on his eyes, tried to tell herself that the bruises on his eyes meant nothing. It didn't work, the assault on her brain by this image of her son could not be warded off by mere logic. Debbie had come up to stand beside her and watched with her as Howard was wheeled past to the ICU, then gently led her back to the group. Where they waited some more. What else could they do?

They spoke more of Amie, of what was to be done, how should they tell her, whether they should they tell her at all. The debate was meaningless, really. Everyone understood that the decision was Debbie's and that she would be the one making it. Earlier, she had quietly pulled Michael aside to talk it over with him. Even as he discussed the pros and cons with her, Michael was marvelling at her composure. Amie's dad had always been the one controlling the family, making the big decisions. Now that had changed, really fast. He had never really seen Debbie in this kind of role. He found it suited her. But he wasn't sure he agreed with her about keeping Amie in the dark. It was her father, didn't she have a right to know? Reluctantly, he agreed to warn her close friends against telling her, just in case she called. They'd have to think of something, though. They couldn't put her off forever.

◆ ◆ ◆

Amie slammed the phone down in frustration. Now she was really annoyed. Why had no one returned her calls? Her dad *always* called her back. She looked at her watch. It was past midnight, which meant that in Toronto it was at least ten in the morning, certainly early enough for people to wake up and check their messages. She'd been calling all day, and hadn't heard a thing. She hated it when she couldn't get in touch with her family, it reminded her that there was an ocean between them. They wouldn't call back now, it was too late. She'd have to wake up early and catch someone then. She set her alarm for five—a little early, but she'd just go for a run—and went to bed.

They were still waiting. Shawna left for a while, returning soon after with her parents. Debbie brought Tyrral and Sonny up to date, something she was getting very used to doing. She should be grateful that it didn't annoy her; she knew that she'd be repeating those details quite a bit in the days to come. Depending, of course, on what happened in that time. Debbie was well aware that there might soon be no need for visitors at this hospital. She tried not to think about that, but one thing the doctors hadn't done was sugarcoat Howard's condition. She supposed she was grateful for that, for having been given the truth. Part of her wished they could have given her hope, instead. The truth hadn't left much room for that. Still, he was alive, and that was better than most others. The doctor had said so himself.

They'd relocated from the OR to another waiting room off the ICU after Howard was moved. Their new room was quieter, darker, with plush couches and chairs that seemed designed for long hours. The odd lamp cast a muted yellow glow. It was fully enclosed, with only a small doorway linking it to the turmoil on the ward outside. There was a different kind of turmoil reserved for this room. Debbie was glad to be away from the bank of orange chairs across from the nursing station, with its out-of-date *Reader's Digest*s and garish fluorescent lighting and sick and needy patients being ferried to and fro. It was a lovely room, comfortable and still, but that didn't change its purpose. It was still a waiting room, for people who could do nothing more than worry, and wait, and mourn.

Debbie looked over at Tyrral and Sonny sitting with their four daughters, and felt a sudden stab of jealousy. When all was said and done, they could go home and know that they still had a family. Debbie had a husband close to death, a daughter across the world, and another daughter whose face had been frozen in the same tearful, frightened expression since this whole ordeal had begun yesterday evening. Yesterday evening—it hadn't even been a day. Debbie felt like she'd aged years in the past twenty hours. She looked over at her sister-in-law's family again, and looked at their faces. Fear, and worry, on all of them. Poor Shawna and Stephen looked lost, and Jill looked haggard and worn. Debbie suddenly realized that Jill had been there with them since 6:30 this morning. No one would be going home unaffected by this.

And then, finally, they were allowed to see Howie. Another doctor had come into the ICU, another neurosurgeon. Dr. Lozano had been the doctor who had arranged Howard's original transfer from the Sinai to the Western, had been the one who had assembled the team that had uncorked Howard's brain. He informed them that Dr. Rocket was in stable condition under intensive care and could now receive a few visitors. He had been conscious intermittently. They were doing all they could. They would have to wait and see. And he had taken Dana and Debbie to see his patient.

They passed out of the cool sanctuary of the waiting room and into the busy hall where nurses in blue and orderlies in pink and doctors in white scurried back and forth with clipboards and IVs. Then they turned left through a broad curtained doorway into the Intensive Care Unit. It was a large room, open, with about eight beds surrounded by tubes and machines and monitors. Doctors and nurses tended to the bodies lying prone on the beds. One of those bodies was Howard.

Dana and Debbie drew closer to the bed, gingerly, as though any stray movement would upset the delicate balance needed by the network of life-saving appliances around him to keep him alive. Howard seemed to be hooked up to every machine in the room. There was a monitor for his heart and for his breathing. Liquid dripped in measured intervals from a plastic bag through an intravenous tube into his arm. Catheters snaked around him so that they couldn't tell where the tubes were going or where they were coming from. And at the center of this vast tangle of tubes and wires was Howard, pale and still.

Dana and Debbie had both seen him, but the shock was still there as they saw the livid bruises ringing his eyes, dark and angry against the pallor of his skin. They could see the faint rise and fall of his chest as his body laboured over each breath, in time with the beeps of the machines monitoring him. Otherwise, he was motionless. Dana still couldn't believe this was her father. Debbie still couldn't believe any of it. How far they had come in this one endless day.

They approached him on the right, recalling the effect the stroke had had on his left side. Gently, Dana reached out to take his hand, and thought she felt a faint pressure in return.

"Howie ... Howie, honey, it's Debbie, and Dana. We're here for you, we're all here for you." Debbie searched his face for signs of awareness, and thought she saw an eyelid flicker. Her heart seized. "Everybody's so proud of you, you're doing so well."

"Hi, Dad. It's Dana, I love you so much, you're going to get better, you're already getting better." Her voice quavered a bit, but it was warm and reassuring and full of love.

Howard tried to focus in the direction of the voices, but he couldn't see them. He pressed against Dana with his good hand again, to let her know he loved her, too, and that he was okay. He heard her say *dad fight a hundred percent, you always fight a hundred percent*, and he tried to tell her that he was trying. But he couldn't speak. He could move, barely, and he tried to show them that he understood, with the right side of his body.

It broke Dana's heart to see him like this. She knew he was in there, fighting to get out, pushing and pushing against whatever it was that was holding him back. She saw it in his struggle to raise his eyelids, felt it in the pressure from his hand. She leaned over and put her hands on his face, letting him feel the life and the love from her touch. She was crying now, again. Debbie had a hand on Dana's shoulder and the other in Howard's, and together they made an unbroken circle.

There was a sound behind them. Tyrral and Marsha were there, and Debbie remembered that there were many others who had the right to see Howie. Gently she led Dana back and motioned Howard's sisters forward.

Tyrral had needed to go in with someone else. She was afraid—not only for him, but *of* him, of the unknown he represented. She was afraid to touch him, lest she do something to make him worse, afraid of anything she knew so little about. She was the eldest, but she had always looked to Howard as being "there" if they needed him. Suddenly, *he* was needy, very needy. It was something she wasn't used to. She and Marsha held hands as they approached their brother.

Oh God, he was a mess. Tyrral felt herself becoming afraid again. He looked all blue, and battered. She couldn't tell if he knew they were there, he was so still. Then she looked at the monitors, and saw his heart rate and blood pressure go up. Maybe he did know. She looked closer at his eyes. They seemed tiny, and heavily glazed, and seemed to look out blankly and unseeing.

"I feel like he can't see us," she whispered to Marsha. "Do you think he knows we're here?" Marsha gave her hand a squeeze and moved to Howard's side, Tyrral following hesitantly.

"Howard, it's Marsha and Tyrral. We're here for you." Marsha searched for something more to say, but found she could only take her brother's hand. God, why could you find nothing intelligent to say when someone was this ill? Tyrral was tongue-tied.

Howard heard his sisters somewhere above him and was so glad to hear their voices. He felt his eyes fill with tears, overwhelmed. His family ... his whole family was there. And he was alive. He was so lucky. He wished he could tell them so. Then he realized that his whole family wasn't there... *Amie ... Risa...* where was his other sister? He tried very hard to ask, sounding the word out carefully with his lips.

Marsha and Tyrral were overcome with emotion at the sight of their brother crying helplessly in that hospital bed. They cried with him, holding his hands and saying his name over and over. They promised to bring Risa. Soon, Howie, soon.

Through the haze, Howard heard them leave, and then Debbie and Dana were back, with somebody else. He heard his mother's voice and wanted to cry again, and then she receded and he heard a voice saying *hi Uncle Howie it's Missy* and then Shawna and Steven were there telling him they loved him, and he loved them, too. Then Jennifer was beside him and Howard tried to tell her to go on with business as usual and motioned to Jennifer that she shouldn't worry. Then he heard Debbie say *Kenny's here* and his friend gripped him tightly and Michael and Michael were there and he heard a voice ask if he wanted Amie to come home. He wanted to say *yes* but couldn't speak so he tried to nod and he hoped they understood. All this was very tiring, and though he wanted to stay with his family, he was so tired, so he struggled to say goodbye and slipped back into sleep.

◆   ◆   ◆

Michael went back to the ICU and straight to Debbie.

"Amie has to be here," he said. She looked at him, surprised. "It's unfair, Debbie. Amie would never forgive us if— God forbid ... she would want to be here." His voice softened. "Howard wants her here, too. You know he does." It was ridiculous. They had to tell Amie.

"Michael, I know," said Debbie. "But she's all alone there, you know that. How can we leave her to deal with this all alone?"

"We won't, and she won't," he said. "I'll go to Tokyo and get her."

She looked at him for a moment. "Thank you," she said.

The Living Shivah

It had been that easy. The decision that had been weighing on her had been made. Amie would come home, and she wouldn't be forced to do it alone. Michael would leave on the next available flight to Tokyo, and would bring Amie straight back. She hoped they would have something promising to return to.

Debbie had wanted to be sure. Part of her wanted to believe that there was no need to bring Amie home, that by the time she got here everything would be fine. So she had asked Dr. Lozano what he thought. She said, "Our daughter is in Japan," and had looked at him questioningly. He had simply said, "If it were my father, I'd want to be here."

Michael called Amie in Japan, from the hospital. She answered on the first ring. "Hello?"

Michael tried to keep his tone light. "Surprise!"

"Michael, hi!" He heard her tone change, knew she had been expecting someone else. In spite of all that was going on, Michael was suddenly happy, hearing her voice. He missed her a lot. This was going to be difficult.

"Amie, I've got great news. Most of my classes this week have been cancelled. It's perfect timing. I'm coming to see you!" How he wished that were true.

"Michael, that's fantastic!" And it was. She was lonely in Japan. She didn't really like her program, as interesting as an MBA was, she missed her family and her friends and her life.

And Michael. She was so happy she almost forgot about what had been troubling her earlier. Almost.

"I'll be on the first plane out tomorrow morning, which means I should be there late Sunday night, or Monday morning, your time."

"I'm so excited you're coming, this is perfect timing. I've been feeling kind a little alone lately. I haven't spoken to anyone in ages." His heart ached for her, she sounded so forlorn. "I've been trying to reach my dad since Friday, and nobody's called me back. Usually someone calls me back."

He hated misleading her about this, but in this case the end justified the means. "I'm sure it's nothing, Amie. You know how busy your dad gets, he told me last week that things were getting pretty crazy. The weekend's not even half over for us— I'm sure you'll speak to someone soon."

She sighed. Of course, he was right, she was overreacting. "You're right, but I was just ... worried. I called my Auntie Shelly this morning, my mom's sister, to find out if anything was going on." Michael had already known this. Shelly had told Debbie.

"What did she have to say?" *The end justified the means. The end justified the means.*

"Oh, that everything was fine, what else? I'd just like to hear for myself." She brightened. "I'm so glad you're coming, Michael."

Michael searched her voice for a hint of suspicion, and detected none. He felt another twinge of guilt. "I'm glad too, Amie. I'll see you soon." And he hung up, hoping he was doing the right thing.

◆　◆　◆

Debbie called her a little later, finally. It was so good to talk to her daughter. Amie had been so relieved to have finally

heard from someone that she accepted Debbie's vague expla-
nation without question.

"Guess what, Mom, Michael's coming! Isn't that great?"
Her daughter sounded so happy. If she only knew.

"That's wonderful, honey." She couldn't think of anything
else to say. What else could she possibly say?

"Mom?" Amie's voice held concern, now. Had she betrayed anything? Damn! "Mom, is everything okay?"

Debbie forced a cheerful note into her voice. She hated
this. "Everything's fine, sweetheart. I'm sorry we didn't get
back to you, we'll try not to get our signals crossed again. Your
dad's been busy."

"Well, tell him to squeeze me in somewhere. I miss him.
How are Sheba and Humphrey?"

Relief. A change of subject. "They're fine, hyperactive as
usual."

Amie laughed. "Just like Dad, I'm sure. Tell him to call
me, okay, Mom?"

Debbie closed her eyes. "Okay, honey. I love you, Amie."

"You too, Mom. Bye."

Their daughter was coming home. She went to tell Howie.

With that situation resolved, they were back to waiting. Nothing much happened in the next twenty-four hours; except that
Howard lived. It was all he had to do. They turned to the doctors, who had said that the first twenty-four hours would be
critical. The doctors told them that Howard was lucky to be alive,
and that they would know more after forty-eight hours. There
wasn't enough known about basilar strokes to be able to predict
his chances just yet. All they could do was wait. For a change.

The crowd in the ICU had swelled yet again. Howard's sister Risa had arrived with her husband, and Uncle Art had come to join the vigil for his nephew. More of Howard's friends were arriving; word of his stroke had trickled throughout the community, as bad news always does. Brian Price had heard at a wedding, and gone straight to the hospital in his tuxedo. Shelly Little had come to the hospital immediately, feeling disoriented himself from the news. Murray Belzberg came on Sunday, wishing he'd never invited Howard to join him in a casual football game. Kenny was still there, joined by his fiancée Kathy. Helen's husband Harry Price, by coincidence the uncle of Brian, sat quietly with his wife as she waited for news of her son.

They were a group of about fifteen to twenty strong at any given moment, filling the ICU with their presence. Theirs was a large family, and they were discovering that they dealt with common tragedy by coming together. They'd always been close, but this was different from bat mitzvahs and seders and brunches. This was sustained and intense and in very close quarters, and they were rediscovering themselves as a family in that room.

They passed the hours in the ICU, quietly reminiscing about Howard. The stories flowed easily among them, and there was much laughter amid the worry and the fear. Sometimes the nurses would have to ask them to keep it down. The core members of the family were reluctant to leave the ward, preferring to eat take-out in the room they were quickly taking over. Visitors brought more food in—they were a large family, and Jewish, so it was natural that they would seek to be well fed. Flowers and cards poured in as news of Howard's stroke spread. It seemed that people, knowing that there was little they could do for Howard now, were trying to alleviate the pain felt by those around him, in whatever small way they could. Debbie was grateful, and made sure the extra flowers were distributed throughout the ward. There was no one in that place who couldn't use some cheering up.

The nurses accepted the flowers gratefully, and would occasionally nosh with the family, who had lots of snacks to spare. Among themselves they wondered who this Howard Rocket was to command such a following, such an outpouring of hope and good wishes. Was he someone famous? They'd never heard of him, but obviously a lot of other people had.

It certainly helped to have people around who cared, Debbie reflected. It took some of the helpless wondering out of waiting. Herself, she wasn't used to snacking in the middle of the day, but if there was ever a time for comfort food, it was now. She had assumed the mantle of control now, and she had forced herself to live up to it. Although she'd spent the first day in sweats, she'd had some decent clothes brought over and had forced herself to get it together. Putting on lipstick and pulling her hair neatly back helped her get a sense of routine, of normalcy, which she desperately needed to avoid falling apart altogether. She couldn't allow herself that; there was too much she had to do.

Risa wasn't sure how she felt about any of this, hadn't been ever since she was awakened in Bracebridge by the call summoning her back to Toronto. Absurd that she should feel so ill at ease among her own family, but there it was. Maybe it was because she was feeling so ambivalent about Howard right now. She'd always been proud of her brother and the success that he had achieved by himself, but she had never related to his preoccupation with power and money. She herself had never been part of that milieu; not that she was complaining, she had done the best she could and she was proud of the stability she'd built up for herself. She hadn't had it easy, what with the divorce and all, but she was happy with her new husband and her children and the values and the life they shared.

She had drifted from Howard and her family since her remarriage; but mostly from Howard. They just weren't on the same wavelength, and a space had ballooned between them over the past few years. It was bound to happen, anyway, in a family as big as this one—how could you possibly be close with everyone? There weren't enough hours in the day. No, she couldn't pretend that things were peachy-keen between Howard and herself when they'd both allowed themselves to move slowly but decisively away from each other.

Which was the reason she was having so much trouble today. Yes, he was her brother, before and after and besides all else. But she hadn't spoken to him in over six months, and there were those feelings to deal with. This was why she hadn't gone straight to the hospital from the cottage, going home instead to unpack and to tell her kids personally about their uncle. She'd needed more time to prepare herself, room to think and figure things out. She had walked into her house like an automaton, feeling no emotion, unpacking and then driving to the hospital. Mentally, she could appreciate what had happened, how close to death he was hovering. Emotionally though, she was disengaged. She couldn't help it.

She'd arrived at the hospital late. No, not late, just later than everybody else. They'd all been in to see him by now. Apparently he'd been calling for her, and she'd felt something when she heard that, she knew.

Then she'd left her family, and gone to the ICU to see her

brother, her eyes taking in the hospital-blue disarray of that room with its medical accoutrements and sickly, bedridden figures. She found her brother among them, lying motionless within the chaos of the room. She approached his bed, slowly, then rested her hand lightly atop the covers. He didn't stir. *Poor, poor Howard,* she thought, *with all your fortune, your power, your good looks, it comes to this.* She wondered at the irony of it all. Abruptly she turned away from the bed. She couldn't look at him like that anymore, not after six months. She walked out of the ICU, back toward the family. Behind her, Howard didn't stir.

◆　◆　◆

They were easing into life in the ICU. Out of chaos had come a sense of routine, keeping everyone sane and somewhat diverted. For the most part, real life had not yet encroached on the inhabitants of that little room; the rigors and responsibilities of the everyday could still be put off, for a little while longer.

The focus was shifting subtly from despair to hope as the hours passed and Howard remained stable. Although the doctors were unable to make any firm predictions, Howard was alive, sometimes even conscious, and that was enough for them.

It was almost enough for Dana. She took comfort in the fact that her father was alive, but there was so much more at stake. They didn't know if he would see or speak again, or if he would ever be able to move from that bed. The idea of her father as anything but the dynamic, vibrant figure she'd always looked up to was unthinkable, and she feared that. She was suddenly superstitious, and found herself talking to God often during the day, silently negotiating for her father's full recovery. She knew that if anyone could beat the odds, it was her father, and she knew he was there inside that feeble body, fighting. Fighting to hang on and come back to the life he loved. She would sit beside him, holding his hand and telling him how much he was loved, and needed. She would know from the monitor pulsing above his bed that he was hearing every word.

She developed an insatiable curiosity about all the medical aspects of his case, and constantly plied Dr. Hu with questions about her father's condition and the treatment he had undergone.

"What happens to the areas of the brain that had no blood during the twelve hours that my father's basilar artery was blocked?" she asked.

"Brain tissue that is deprived of blood eventually dies," Dr. Hu explained. "Areas like this are called 'infarcts.' Once brain cells are dead they are useless, and simply melt away, leaving a space. Brain cells cannot be replaced."

"What happens to the dye that you injected into my father's bloodstream in order to pinpoint the clot?"

"It gets excreted by the kidneys. Harmless. Probably all gone by now."

Dana would listen intently and carefully store this new knowledge away in her mind. Dr. Hu came by one afternoon with a medical textbook, and she read, and memorized. She needed to know as much as she could.

Around the same time, Michael shifted in his sleep aboard a plane hurtling through the sky on its way to Tokyo.

◆   ◆   ◆

Consciousness sometimes seeped into Howard through the haze that enveloped him. He couldn't see and he couldn't speak, but he could sense the presence of his family and friends around him, and he could hear their voices floating above him when they spoke. He liked having those floating voices anchored to him by a hand or an embrace. When the disembodied voices seemed too far away, he would try with his right side to communicate with visitors. He'd thumped on his chest before Shawna and Stephen, and they'd understood that he'd wanted to hug them, to show them the strength in his good arm. At that point, Shawna and Stephen hadn't known who was comforting whom.

In fact, Howard didn't feel like he needed comforting. He was not afraid, hadn't been since they'd wheeled him from an ambulance into the emergency room of the Sinai. He knew everything would be okay, which was what made it so easy for him to slip back into the welcoming haze whenever it engulfed him again.

Debbie was exhausted. She'd been sleeping at the hospital, in the ICU. She knew every nook and cranny of that God-awful room. It was the new family headquarters, she thought wryly. She'd been keeping it together, though, despite her fatigue. She'd had a lot of help in that. She had one Michael to thank for helping her resolve the dilemma about Amie, and the other Michael to thank for helping Dana cope with this nightmare. The calm, easy confidence radiated by Michael Kalles made it very hard to doubt that he had everything under control. It seemed to comfort Dana, and for that Debbie was grateful.

She had received a lot of support from their friends, too. After changing out of his tux, Brian Price showed up at 7 AM

the next morning as Debbie woke up, bearing steaming, refreshing coffee. He did so the next morning, too. Together
they'd go and see Howie, talking to him as the machines
hummed in the background. Their close friends Michael and
Lillian Winton were ICU fixtures as well. Lillian was a phar-
macist, and offered readily accessible knowledge about
Howard's medications and condition. Michael had gone to university with Howard, and the two had become close when
Michael had taken over Tridont's legal work in the mid-eight-
ies. He'd been badly shaken after seeing Howard. He hadn't
been ready for what he saw. Had any of them?

The doctors were helpful and attentive, but could offer no
more real hope. Basilar thrombosis was too rare to be able to
gauge Howard's progress. Or his prognosis. They'd been fairly
blunt about the probability of damage. Permanent damage. Debbie
had no idea of what had gone on in Howard's brain, really. She
knew that her husband was basically at rock bottom now, and
that they couldn't tell her if he'd ever get better. That translated
into a very different kind of life for them all in the future. Just
thinking about it exhausted her. She could only get through this
crisis minute by minute. At least now he was stable. At least he
wasn't getting worse.

He got worse. Howard had a feeding tube in his mouth,
but his gag reflex wasn't functioning properly. The doctors
feared that fluid might drip down and fill his lungs. They had
no choice but to perform a tracheostomy on Howard, inserting
a tube through a hole in his throat just below his Adam's apple.
The tube would inhibit normal breathing, speaking and swallowing functions. The doctors weren't sure how temporary it

would be. Yet another tube to hook Howard up to the medical machinery of neurointensive care. It was a downward slide.

As was the pneumonia. Fluid collected in his lungs, despite preventive measures. His every breath sounded thin, wheezy. Another medication was added to the list. Another sickness to fight against. The doctors were very guarded, soberly reminding the family that they wouldn't know much until he'd made it to seventy-two hours. Forty-eight simply wasn't enough, not for a basilar stroke. They'd just have to wait. Again.

The hours seemed to melt away, but slowly. They tried not to watch the clock; time was no longer measured in minutes and hours, but in Howard's breathing, or by the beat of his pulse. He held on to life in that room that was for people more dead than alive, where the work of machines produced vital signs that weren't vital at all. Occasionally one of the family would go in and stand quietly by his side, looking down at the ashen face and wondering how deeply the spirit of their Howie was buried inside the inert form on the bed. Later, they would return to the waiting room a little more subdued, until the warmth of the family drew them out and reminded them that they, at least, were still alive.

Beyond the
Hundredth Hour

Visiting was now cut back. Howard needed to recuperate in the unbroken calm of the ICU, to be focused completely on recovery. They could not risk having him roused to emotional intensity and whatever internal upheaval might ensue. Dr. Lozano had seen that Howard's effort to stay awake for his visitors was exhausting him. His patient would not best cling to life that way.

Debbie was an unbending gatekeeper, granting admittance sparingly to her husband's side. But it didn't matter; the crowd in the ICU remained the same. They were there as much for each other as for the man lying in a room beyond. The comfort of the ICU routine provided a soothing counterpart to the horror of their unspoken fears.

Howard's family and friends became acquainted, then involved, with other ICU families. As the hours crawled past in the waiting room, they exchanged hospital résumés and acknowledged their unwilling membership in the same community. Theirs were shared triumphs and moments of sadness in that space as they hoped and waited for news, any news. Some weepy faces would suddenly be gone, and others appeared. They were often reminded that the ICU was a place that didn't see many happy endings.

It was a reminder that echoed often in the empty hours of waiting.

◆   ◆   ◆

Michael was awakened by the soft thump of the aircraft touching the tarmac. He was twisted awkwardly in his seat, dimly aware of a tingling foot and an aching neck. He unwound his body and felt his muscles creak in protest. It was going to be a long, long day.

As soon as the plane had taxied to a stop, Michael grabbed his bag and was off—a relief after eighteen hours. He knew he'd be back at this airport in another eighteen hours for a second uncomfortable journey across the sky, back to Toronto and, he hoped, good news. But right now he had to put a smile on his face for Amie, who thought they were about to spend a carefree, romantic week together in Tokyo. He had to look the part.

He could see her waiting for him outside the arrival gate, excited and unsuspecting. As hard as the next few minutes were going to be, he was glad that he wasn't going to have to lie to her much longer. He realized that he'd unconsciously slowed his pace, and that other passengers had overtaken him and were already outside the gate. There was no use making this harder than it had to be; he might as well get it over with immediately. He reluctantly quickened his pace.

Amie could see him coming along the corridor, and she felt a rush of happiness. She was so excited, it had been too long and she had felt too isolated from her life back home. She couldn't wait to give Michael her biggest hug. She still couldn't believe he had been able to come. God, she was so lucky! She pushed impatiently closer to the gate and saw him hurrying toward her, and then there he was and she was enveloped in the comfort of one of his hugs and she was so happy that for some bizarre reason she thought she might cry.

Michael was just happy to hold on to her for a moment

that almost felt like normal. Everything else aside, it was so great to see her. He wished he could just keep the everything else aside. But, after all, he had a reason for being there.

Amie was looking at him. "Michael," she said slowly, as if trying to understand something, "why is your bag so small?" He looked down at his little travel shoulder bag, and didn't have an answer.

Amie wasn't listening, anyway. Things were coming together in her mind.

You know how busy your dad gets.

No one had returned her calls.

Everything's fine, sweetheart, we'll try not to get our signals crossed again.

Her dad *always* returned her calls.

Your dad's been busy.

Her dad was *never* that busy.

Tell him to call me, okay, Mom?

He hadn't called.

"Michael," she said, "what's wrong with my father?"

◆　◆　◆

Debbie checked her watch again. It had become a nervous habit over the last hour, when she knew Michael was to have landed in Tokyo. She'd given him specific instructions to have Amie call her immediately, at the hospital. She wanted to be the one to tell Amie about her father.

Not much had changed since Michael had taken off yesterday. Thank God, anything could happen in eighteen hours. Now nineteen, almost. She checked her watch again. Howard was still on the brink, hovering somewhere between consciousness and darkness. She would sit with him and talk to him quietly, holding his hand and telling him about all the people who were there for him in the waiting room. Sometimes she would see a flicker of response, feel a gentle pressure from his right hand. Only from his right, though. Howard was still paralyzed on his left side.

The phone rang. She lifted the receiver before it could ring twice. "Amie?"

"Mom?" Her daughter was sobbing at the other end, somewhere across the world. Shock. Worry. Fear. "Is he okay?"

Debbie felt her own tears well up, stilled the quaver in her own voice. She felt relief at finally being honest with her daughter. "He's stable, sweetheart. The doctors are doing all they can."

"I'm coming home, Mom. I should be there now." Debbie felt a stab of guilt, but right now Amie was too anxious to be angry. And she needed some answers. "What are his chances? Is he going to ... will he be okay?"

Debbie sighed. Now was the time to be honest. "Well, he lived through the night."

Amie was stunned. Michael had comforted her, assuring her that her dad was a fighter, that he was going to be fine. *Living* she had taken for granted. It appeared that nothing could be taken for granted any more. Life. Health. Family.

"How badly has it affected his brain?" Would there be permanent damage? Would he walk again? Had she lost forever the father she knew? The questions came in a rush, in a panic, so quickly and so many that she couldn't ask them all.

"Amie, there's nothing conclusive I can tell you right now except that he's alive. The first three days are the critical period and he's almost through it. His chances increase dramatically once he reaches seventy-two hours."

The words were hopeful, but Amie found little comfort in

statistics. She needed to be there, to direct the force of her own vitality toward her father. Three days had never seemed like much time to her before, but suddenly each hour she had missed felt like a blow. And she couldn't waste any more.

Unfortunately, she would have to. She'd wanted to leave as soon as Michael told her, but there were no flights home until the next afternoon. Did anyone think she couldn't handle being there for her father when he needed her the most? He'd brought her up to do better than that. She'd cancel an exam, hunt down her passport, settle up, wind down, whatever. She'd do what was needed to fill the time—but absolutely nothing would keep her off that first flight out of Tokyo.

Her mother was apologizing for not telling her sooner. It mattered, but not right now.

"Tell Dad I love him, Mom, and tell him I'm on my way home."

A relief. Amie was coming home. Now that the wheels were in motion, she just wanted her daughter here, now. Because Howard wasn't getting any better. In fact, the longer he remained in his transient state, the less likely it was that he was going to recover. Reality was hitting hard, as Debbie forced herself to confront the possibilities that lay in the future. He couldn't talk. He couldn't move. He couldn't see. She didn't even know if he could breathe without being hooked up to a machine. This was what had become of her husband. And he might not get better.

Debbie sat with her family while Amie, halfway around the world, prepared to come home. And the clock moved silently past seventy-two hours as Howard lay unmoving and unchanged.

◆ ◆ ◆

Rose Ouellet was driving, taking the highway between Grimsby and Toronto as fast as the speed limit would allow. Right now the straight expanse of road beyond the dashboard was the only thing keeping her under control. She gripped the steering wheel, instinctively applying a little more pressure to the accelerator. She had to get to Howard.

That was all that had been on her mind since she got the phone call late that afternoon, from an old friend she'd worked with during her Tridont days. Listening politely as she chattered on. Apologizing for having to be the one to tell her. Asking her if she was sitting down. Telling her about Howard.

After that came a blur of tears and confusion, of trying to figure out who to call and where to look. Pulling out faded cards from the Rolodex, old files from working days. Calling around, leaving messages, then calling the hospitals until she found out where he was. Then into the car, and off.

They had told her at the hospital that he was in intensive care and that she wouldn't be able to see him. She didn't care. She would just stand near the elevator until she saw someone who could tell her how he was. She hadn't seen or spoken to Howard for two years, but she had certainly thought of him. Two years was a long time. There wasn't any problem between them, but she had been avoiding him, she knew. She had worked closely with Howard back at Tridont, and he had invited her to work with him again on his latest project. She'd been quite happy as a housewife, but she found herself getting excited, as she always did. He'd always been able to get her as motivated about any of his ideas as if they were her own. He'd given her the literature, explained it to her, and asked her to think about it.

She had thought about it. And the more she thought, the more she couldn't help remembering how exciting it was to work with Howard. They'd put in fourteen years together at Tridont, and they'd both worked hard at a job they loved. She'd been lucky, falling into her position there. But then again, he'd also been lucky. Not everyone could have kept up with him. She wasn't sure she could do it again, but she found herself tempted to try.

Howard had told her that nothing would be happening for at least six months, that they were still seeking approval from the proper authorities, and that he'd be in touch with her when things were rolling. That had been in May, when she had been making plans to go back to school. She decided to wait for Howard to call her, hoping that by the time he did she'd be knee deep in textbooks and exams. It would be easier than trying to resist him.

The six months had come and gone, and Rose had been relieved. Howard had not called. No big decisions to make, after all. Then a year passed, and Rose heard the rumor that she and Howard would be working together again. She felt guilty, as though she'd let him down or embarrassed him some-how. She put off calling him, even to say hello.

The year stretched into two, and Rose continued with her schooling and her life. Howard still hadn't called, and Rose was still too nervous to call him. It was silly, but she was afraid that he was angry with her. She couldn't bear having Howard reject her. She loved him like a brother.

Now he was in the hospital, and they'd lost two precious years, and her silly anxieties didn't seem that important any more.

She finally reached the hospital and started toward the ICU. She knew it was family only, and that was okay. It was enough just to be near, to show Howard and his family her support. She followed the signs directing her to the ICU and tentatively approached the waiting room, half-expecting to be stopped. She hesitated, hearing hushed voices down the corridor, not wanting to intrude. Suddenly Howard's sister Marsha walked out of the waiting room, and Rose froze. Marsha was looking at her. *Oh, my God, she sees me,* she thought in panic. *Am I intruding? Will she ask me to leave? Does she even know who I am?*

Marsha stepped toward Rose, and wrapped her arms around her, holding her tightly. "It will be all right," she said, giving Rose a squeeze. She took Rose by the hand and led her into the waiting room.

"Look, everyone. Look who's here." And suddenly Rose was facing Howard's family, and they greeted her with warmth, and she was reassured that perhaps it really was okay that she was there. Then Debbie came over to Rose and hugged her, and that was when Rose started crying again and found that she could not stop.

Debbie gently led Rose to a bank of chairs down the hall, holding her hands while their old friend wept.

"I'm sorry, Debbie," she managed after a while. "I just found out this afternoon, and I had to come right over." Rose hesitated, wanting to know more but afraid to ask.

Debbie understood. After four days of fielding anxious visitors she was used to reading their unspoken signals. "It's okay, Rose, Howard would be thrilled to know that you are here. He's stable right now, and we've made it past the first seventy-two hours. Apparently that's a good sign, but he hasn't improved at all. We're all praying for him, and the doctors are doing all they can. You know Howard's a fighter. He'll pull through." Rose did know. However weakened Howard was, he had a core of stubbornness and tenacity that no affliction could touch. That knowledge gave her a small measure of comfort.

"Rose." She looked up, and Brian Price was standing there. Another old friend. So many memories coming so unexpectedly. She hugged Brian and his wife, Gilda, and hoped that Howard could somehow sense the warmth that had collected here because of him.

Debbie was talking to someone from intensive care. She nodded, and came back over to them. "They'll let Howard have a few visitors right now. Rose, do you want to go in with Brian to see Howard?" Rose tried to respond, but found her tears welling up again. She nodded, so grateful that they understood how she felt.

Since she had left the work force, Rose had volunteered with her local palliative care unit, assisting terminally ill people, offering them quiet company in the last few months of their lives, providing what comfort she could. She had watched her patients wither away under the onslaught of disease, stayed with them as they deteriorated, had been with people at the moment they died. But none of that had prepared her to see Howard.

He looked closer to death than anyone she had ever seen. And she knew he was dying, even as she went over to him and took his hand and kissed his cheek and told him that she loved him. He lay there, unresponsive and unseeing, seeming to gaze vacantly through her, and she knew he was dying. Howard was dying.

It was dark where Howard was, and quiet. He couldn't remember how long he'd been there, but it didn't seem to matter. The harsh lights of the emergency room seemed like a very long time ago, far away from where he was now. He felt peaceful and unafraid.

Sometimes he could hear voices swimming high above him, but they didn't seem to matter anymore, either. He was cocooned in a sweet hazy darkness on all sides, and it was a warmth he didn't want to leave. But now it was quiet and the voices had faded into the mist, and he was alone.

And now the darkness seemed to shift, to take shape away from the mist that enclosed him. He felt as though the darkness was tunnelling away from him, leading him out of his cocoon toward something else. And he felt that he was standing upright, and moving forward through the tunnel. And he saw that at the end of the tunnel was a golden light, shimmery and hazy and warm, and welcoming. And then the tunnel felt less like a tunnel than an open space bounded by the light, and he was in that space facing the light directly. Through the melting, shimmering haze he could see figures, gray and indistinct, moving behind the light. He sensed that they shared the warmth that came from the light. He looked for his father among the gray shadows, but could not see him. And suddenly he was afraid, because he was alone on his side of the light, alone in the gray nothingness at the end of the tunnel, and no one had come to greet him or tell him where he was. He was alone, and the light beckoned, and then he was running away, away from the light and the warmth and the shadows, away from a place where he felt himself alone, away. And as he moved back down the tunnel and away from the light, he felt himself moving toward the voices that had reached down to him through the fog, and he was reaching up to them, moving faster and faster through the fog to get to them, reaching out toward the voices, and he was moving faster and faster and he felt himself fall backward, and he was falling, falling and then he was lying on his back and looking up and that was when he saw Rose and Brian.

Waking

Outside, the traffic on Bathurst Street was navigating the first real snowfall of the year. People clad in scarves, gloves and boots hurried by in the morning rush hour, dodging the puddles of slush beginning to form. The sun was out, but still their breath hung briefly in the air, suspended in a frosty cloud before dissolving into the crisp chill of the November morning. No one paused to take in the sunshine or breathe in the cool of early winter. There wasn't time. It was rush hour, after all.

Above, in a room on the fifth floor of Toronto Western Hospital, someone was looking out at the sunshine. It was a small room, private and functional, with the barest of furnishings surrounding the bed in its center. An intravenous bag dripped slowly as monitors hummed in the background. A jungle of flowers, plants, balloons and baskets festooned the room, filling it with color and brightness and life, catching the light of the morning sun slanting through the window. From his hospital bed in the middle of the room, Howard Rocket looked out the window at the sun and was glad.

It was great to be alive. Despite the fact that he could not speak, stand, or move one-half of his body, Howard considered himself to be one of the luckiest guys around. Here he was, finally out of the ICU, still around after a massive stroke. Still around to see sunshine, to watch the snow falling. Still around to see the world and be a part of it. Awake. *Alive.*

It had been pretty close, he knew that now. Funny, even when he'd been at his worst he'd never really been afraid. Except of the light. It had been so welcoming, so warm, but he had been afraid that he would like it too much. That he would stay. He didn't know where or what that place was, but he had known he wasn't ready to be a permanent resident. So he ran away, and the next thing he knew he was seeing Rose and Brian.

He hadn't realized it at the time, but that had been big news. The next thing he'd known there were nurses and doctors surrounding him and Debbie and Dana had been there, crying and laughing and hugging him. He was happy, too, that he was getting better, but he wasn't surprised; it had never occurred to him that he wouldn't.

Then he'd tried to hug them back, but could only lift his right arm. And he knew he wasn't quite all better. Yet.

Howard heard the quiet scrape of his door being opened, and turned his head from the window to watch his daughter walk in. She came over and gave him a kiss on the forehead, then sat down beside him and took his hand.

"Morning, Daddy. How are you feeling?" He couldn't respond, not verbally. But she could read his answer in his face and in his eyes, and it made her so happy and relieved that she almost didn't care that he couldn't tell her himself. Almost.

She smoothed his hair back from his forehead and put his glasses on for him. There. Now at least he could see properly. Howard's vision hadn't been the greatest even before the stroke, and right now wearing his habitual contacts wasn't possible. He looked so helpless, her father, lying back in bed with those enormous thick-lens glasses perched on his nose. She felt an overwhelming wave of love for him, and the familiar fierce protectiveness washed over her again, renewing her determination to keep him healthy and well. She took his hand again.

"You're looking great this morning, Dad. A lot better. At this rate, you'll be out of here in no time." And it was true. Howard's color was slowly coming back, the grayish tones giving way to shades of peach and rose. Amie remembered how horrified she'd been when she first saw him. It had been so overwhelming, walking into that hospital after the stress and the fear and the worry of the previous twenty-four hours. They'd come straight from the airport to the hospital, not even stopping to phone Debbie to let her know they'd arrived safely. And Amie had walked into the ICU and found her entire family there, her mother and her sister and her aunts, uncles and cousins, the friends that were family and the family that were friends. She'd had to cry then, as she hugged her mother and sister. But she was determined to be strong for her Dad, and that was who she was there to see.

Her mother and sister had led her in to see her father, and she felt the tears coming again. Her father looked so pale, and his skin looked so gray and mottled against the harsh purple bruises under his eyes. But his eyes were open and he was reaching out to her with one arm, and Amie forgot all about being strong as she rushed over to embrace the father she'd so nearly lost. She held on to him, careful of the tube sticking out of his throat, his good arm slung across her back. He was weak, yes, but he was alive. That was all that mattered.

That had been one week ago. In that time, the changes had been enormous. Once Howard had woken up, his condition had improved steadily. Each day he became stronger and more stable, and his dependence on the ICU life-support system decreased. Dr. Lozano was extremely pleased with his progress, and ordered his tracheotomy tube moved from eight to six inches. A good sign. Soon Howard might be breathing on his own. Soon Howard might be doing everything on his own. He was alert and aware, and totally focused on recovery.

It didn't take long before he had outgrown the ICU. Five days after his brain had exploded in a stroke, he was out of intensive care and in a private room on the neurology ward, overlooking a Bathurst Street funeral parlor. The irony had escaped no one, least of all Amie, who lived with the knowledge that she might have flown home for a funeral. She wouldn't have been able to forgive herself for being away when he needed her most. She could barely forgive herself now.

She'd forgiven her family, though, for not telling her. They'd done what they had thought was right. They'd tried to spare her. So they had lied to her, for a while. She tried to not resent them for it, especially now that her dad was doing so well. It was funny, how other people saw you. She knew she was strong inside, so it had never occurred to her that others didn't. Even Michael, who knew her better than anyone. *I guess that's a byproduct of a crisis,* she thought. *You learn that what you thought was true in life can change.* She'd learned more about her own family over the past few days than she'd thought possible. Which was another reason forgiveness came easily.

Besides, now wasn't a time to pick fights. It all seemed so unimportant next to the drama going on in the room on the fifth floor. A flicker in the leg. A twitch in the arm. These were the little milestones that defined her life right now. She smiled at her father, whose gaze had returned to the window and the sunshine. He made getting better look easy.

Getting better was hard work. And it took a long time. Howard was frustrated. He wanted to move and speak and walk and run and live. The doctors shook their heads gravely, said he had to be realistic, that he might not do any of these things again. So what? They were the same people who said he probably wouldn't survive. Well, he'd survived, all right, and he was going to do everything else, too.

But it was hard work getting there. Now that he was stable and out of ICU, the hospital's efforts had moved from keeping him alive to helping him live. He'd started physiotherapy and felt optimistic about his progress. He had two physiotherapists, Debbi and Fidelma, and he looked forward every day to the hours they spent with him. It was difficult, it was frustrating, it was painful, it was slow and it was damn hard work, but it was progress and he loved it. They'd seen him first in the ICU, and continued working with him once he'd moved upstairs to the ward. Dana had looked at their notes, so she knew everything possible about her dad's condition. "Spatially impaired ... no awareness of midline ... left hemiplegia ... unable to sit independently." These were the technical terms for being flat on your back in a hospital bed. He wanted to read what they had to say when he got out of bed and walked out of the hospital. Soon, soon.

Debbie and the girls would watch his therapy, beaming from the sidelines every time he showed an improvement. Sometimes other family or friends would stop in to show their encouragement. Howard was always especially glad to see Kenny Field, who was living proof that physiotherapy worked. Debbi and Fidelma inwardly wondered at the constant stream of Howard's cheerleaders, but were glad to see their patient making some headway. It was funny, their patient couldn't talk, but they could always sense his optimism and excitement during the sessions. In their profession, it was unusual to see that kind of attitude at this stage; most people were still coming to grips with being impaired and hadn't gotten past the "why me?" stage of bitterness and pessimism. They were glad that this one seemed to have left that stage behind. It was certainly helping them do their jobs.

Not being able to speak was driving Howard crazy. The thoughts were tumbling wildly through his head and he was bursting with things he wanted to tell everybody. He'd mouth the words, or try to sign with his good hand. Conversations became guessing games, like they were playing charades and he was always the one up. They'd bought a chalkboard for him to write on, but his motor control wasn't up to it yet, and deciphering his handwriting (never an easy task even before the stroke) took some effort. It was so slow, it drove him nuts. By the time they figured out what he was saying a million other thoughts had come and gone.

Kenny Field helped solve that problem, or at least made communication easier until he got his voice back. He'd gone to the Bay and picked up a "Speak & Spell," a kid's toy Howard hadn't seen since Dana was in diapers. Now he was the one in training and this toy was the communicative link between him and everyone around him. Funny how things evolved. At any rate, between the chalkboard and the Speak & Spell, communication was a lot easier and a lot quicker.

But the one who could always understand him was Dana. She just knew. Maybe it was because she hadn't left his side ever since he got out of ICU. Once he was safe, Dana had finally sensed her fear dissipate. She had felt so helpless, so powerless to help her father, struggling to come to grips with his condition and the machines and the medical terminology and the fact that there was nothing she could do. And the fear had been a constant, trapping her and locking her in with stress and worry and uncertainty. Whenever she had to leave his side in the ICU, she would always look deep into his eyes so she'd know that, God forbid, if she never could again, she'd always have a picture of him burned into her mind. It was the helplessness that had been the worst, knowing that all you can do is simply be there, a warm body taking up space in a waiting room. She had no control. That had chafed the most.

Now things were different. He was stable, he was going to get better, and she was going to help him every step of the way.

So Dana moved in. She was superstitious, she didn't want to leave his side. They'd rolled in a little trundle bed for her, and they were in business. She didn't care about school, or any of the responsibilities of the outside world. Her world was inside this hospital room. And, finally, she was not powerless and she was not helpless. And fear was replaced with hope, and determination.

She became Howard's private nurse. She didn't want him to have to wait for anything. There had been times when he'd touched the call button and there wouldn't be a response for twenty minutes. Well, she had no other duties to attend to. She could look after him. She could be his right arm. Or left, all things considered.

She would fluff his pillows and brush his hair, adjust his bed so he could watch TV or close the curtains so he could sleep. She'd massage his dormant limbs, kneading the muscles back to life. She was brisk and businesslike, cleaning his tracheostomy site, emptying his urinal, sponging him down. She had no problem doing any of these things. She wasn't squeamish in the least. He was her father, for God's sake. He'd done the same for her, once upon a time. She didn't want him to feel embarrassed or ashamed.

Debbie and Amie marvelled at her, at her confidence and

her competence. Both of them had always been queasy types, and both had been known to faint at the sight of blood. But it wasn't so much the squeamishness as the fear of doing something wrong, something to make it worse. How did Dana just know what to do? They would watch her transferring him from bed, hefting him easily and expertly. They'd help her, when she asked, lifting or pushing according to her direction. Getting Howard better was a family affair.

It was an affair for the whole family, who rejoiced in the opportunity to continue bonding under more hopeful circumstances. Between his sisters and their kids, the ward was crawling with visitors. Two daughters, three sisters, twelve nieces, three great-nieces, one great-nephew, a couple of in-laws, a few other odd relations and a whole slew of friends kept Howard entertained and the nurses confused.

The entourage hadn't diminished in the slightest. On the contrary, now that Howard was out of danger, many friends and associates who hadn't wanted to intrude upon the family in the ICU were coming to call. Names from Howard's past. Lorne Frohman, from his Camp Timberlane days. Shelly Bleiman, his old partner. Shelly Little, relieved and a bit less woozy. Sandy Jacobs, an old friend from New York. Barry Taube, a former buddy from forty years ago, now the distinguished Orthodox Rabbi Baruch Taube. Even though Helen had once served him milk and cookies, she was slightly awed. And their rabbi from Beth Sholom Synagogue had been most impressed.

For Howard, it was as emotional as it was wonderful. He was at the center of a complex web of friendship and love, linked and interlinked to all of these people by the enduring span and depth of the years. Sometimes he would have the eerie sense of being a guest at his own funeral. But they were all here to celebrate life and living, especially Howard. Right now, life was the easy part. Living he was working on. Because at the end of the day, all of them could walk out of the hospital.

And he couldn't fully celebrate until he could walk out with them.

Talking

Howard watched the sky streak into morning, the dark gray hues of dusk giving way to light and brightness. He was always up by this time of day, like a little kid, and he loved it. He couldn't help it—watching a new day break always filled him with excitement. To a person who is sick, *morning is a great time*, he thought. *That's when your life can start again. You've made it to another day.*

He looked over at his daughter folded awkwardly into the small hospital trundle bed beside him. She liked to sleep in a little later, always protesting at the early hour. But he knew she was as excited by each new day as he was. He kept looking at her, knowing that if he stared long enough she would eventually wake up. It was seven o'clock and he was impatient for the day to begin.

It wasn't long before Dana opened her eyes. Focusing, she saw her dad's eyes were already open and fixed upon her own, excited and expectant. The glow coming off him was supercharged, energizing Dana with his excitement and her own. God, it was so great to wake up here every day. She felt the same feeling of joy and gratitude that had tucked itself permanently into her heart since her dad had woken up. He was so great. Everything was so great.

Happily leaving behind the trundle bed for another day, Dana got up and opened the blinds wide to let in all the morning light. Her dad was beaming at her. Beaming back, she crossed to the bathroom and got his shaver and toothbrush. A morning ritual: the quick whir of a razor to take care of morning stubble, and a careful regimen of oral hygiene for the man who knew the dangers of neglect. Dana took great pleasure in making her father look totally healthy and well. She'd brush his hair and dab a bit of cologne on his neck, and settle his glasses owlishly on his nose, all the while chatting to him easily.

Chatting *with* him, actually. Even though Howard couldn't speak, their conversations were never one-sided. Howard interacted with his eyes and his face and his good hand, communicating easily with his daughter, who always seemed to know what he meant. He'd motion her to his left side so he'd be forced to work on his inert left limbs. This was a habit he'd gotten into with all his visitors—Howard wouldn't waste a second's opportunity to get well.

And it was taking a lot of seconds. And a lot of minutes, and hours, and days of plain hard work. It would have been unbelievable to him just two weeks ago that he'd want to go for a jog—or even go to the bathroom!—and simply not be able to. And he knew that two weeks ago he himself would have considered the guy in the hospital bed a cripple, pitying his inability to speak and move and eat and breathe at will. Now he knew differently. And he knew he was no cripple. There was no way he was staying in this bed. There was no way he was staying in this hospital. And there was no way he was staying out of life, just when he'd won it back so narrowly. It made the frustration and the pain and the sweat and the work worth it. It would make success that much sweeter.

Howard had no doubt that success would come. Neither did Dana. And today brought them one more step closer to it.

◆ ◆ ◆

Things were slipping into a routine. Dana would have coffee and breakfast while her dad enjoyed the succulent meal offered by the IV. Soon Debbie and Amie would arrive with newspapers and magazines and flowers. Debbie would reel off the list of phone messages from well-wishers. They'd had a VCR hooked up to his television set, and Debbie would bring a selection of tapes for Howard to view. This made for a full morning of family activity.

Two hours every day were allotted to physiotherapy, and Howard worked furiously during those two hours. Such a struggle, just to move his thumb a little! It was like pushing with all his strength against a brick wall—exhausting and futile. But sometimes that wall would give, just a little, and he'd be fired up with hope again, and push even harder.

His family was always there for his therapy. Dana remembered how he'd looked that first day of therapy, a grown man in nothing but a diaper, lying awkwardly on a table because he didn't know how to sit up. She'd been incredulous; how could he not know how to sit? *This is going to be such a long road*, she thought wearily. But already she could see that they had travelled some way along it. He was learning, slowly, and that was great, but there really was no substitute for attitude, and her dad had the best. It was his attitude and his determination and his conviction that would propel him back to health.

They were lucky, too, to have a physiotherapist in the family. Tyrral's daughter Kelli Young had been giving professional consultations ever since the stroke, and positive words from her carried weight. When Howard wasn't in official therapy sessions, Kelli would spend extra time teaching the family how to help him, and Howard how to help himself. Professionally, Kelli had doubts about how much he could recover—she knew the extent of the damage, she'd seen patients who had been in less serious shape still impaired after years and years of therapy. But this was her uncle, and the personal side of her had faith that he'd be able to do it. He certainly wanted it bad enough.

During his other therapy sessions, Debbi and Fidelma were encouraging, and praised his drive and tenacity. They tried to teach him why his body was moving differently now that he was impaired, and how to avoid compensating with his right side, tempting though that might be. They explained where his center of balance was, and why small, controlled movements were far more impressive than large, sloppy ones. Howard listened carefully, and memorized what they told him so that for him, therapy could be a twenty-four hour occurance.

Amie was busy learning, too. A feeling of helplessness lingered in her, left over from her early obliviousness and late arrival. Where Dana had felt helpless because she'd been right there and yet could do nothing, Amie's helplessness came from how stupid and ignorant she'd felt when she finally learned that she'd been gaily cavorting around Tokyo while her father lay dying in a hospital ward thousands of miles away. Suddenly everything she'd done during that time away seemed petty and selfish, and she'd felt the same way. It had all happened without her. She'd meant nothing to the process. She was a non-factor.

At least, that was how she'd felt. Sometimes the helplessness and frustration would build inside her, pushing out from her chest in something very close to pain. She tried to alleviate it now by learning everything she could about her dad's condition. She had gotten a few medical textbooks from the doctors, and when her dad was occupied she would slip out to the nurses' station, reading and studying at the desk there. She wasn't a born nurse like Dana, but she might as well be a doctor for all that she'd learned since she'd been home. She now knew what had happened to her dad, where it had happened, how it had happened and why. She understood in detail how his surgery had progressed and why it had worked, knew what his chances of recovery were and how long it might take.

Everyone had thought she was weak and emotional, but she knew she was the only one who was realistic about her dad's recovery. She shared their optimism about him and his spirit and his will, but she also knew there was a physical body involved whose repair couldn't just be wished for. She asked the doctors questions that she believed her mother and sister hadn't come to terms with, about long-term nursing care and wheelchair accessibility and lifelong dependency. Dr. Lozano had told her that her dad was only one out of four patients he had seen to survive this kind of stroke by this treatment. She understood the significance of statistics. So she kept reading. At least she knew she'd be prepared for whatever else came.

Debbie was too tired to think about the future. She'd become an expert at just getting through the days one at a time. Howard had been asleep for a lot of them. She'd been awake for most.

Thank God for the two Michaels. They'd really demonstrated a commitment to her daughters and the family. As far as she was concerned, they were family now. Michael Wuls had been here for Amie since he'd taken that God-awful round trip to Tokyo. He'd been at the hospital virtually around the clock at the beginning, and he was still logging hospital hours for most days. Amie was on leave from school, but Michael was still in law school, in his all-important second year, which could make or break his employment prospects. He had exams coming up; he should have been at the library. Instead, he'd turned the hospital into his library, sitting with his textbooks in the waiting area or by the window in Howard's room. He'd joke about it, saying that, what's the difference, it was the same fluorescent lighting, but Debbie knew it was a sacrifice, and she appreciated it.

And Michael Kalles, what a crutch he'd been for them all. Howard's optimism was mirrored in Michael, who had remained intensely positive throughout the whole ordeal. He was a lot like Howard, actually—positive and decisive—a doer. That had helped Debbie out, too. One day she'd looked at a calendar and realized that it had been almost two weeks since everything had changed. And she realized with shock that it had been two weeks of not gathering the mail or returning phone calls or dealing with any of the matters that become so habitual in everyday life. The end of the month had come and gone, and they probably owed money all over the city. Michael had taken that burden off her hands, gathering the bills and getting them to the accountant without incident.

But as helpful as Michael was, it wasn't his responsibility, and next month was going to roll around soon enough. Someone had to deal with the practicalities of their lives, and right now Debbie was the best they had. She'd met with the accountant and he'd let her know that they were all right, thank God. She'd honestly had no idea—Howard had always looked after the bills and the finances. She didn't feel shame or embarrassment about that fact—they'd worked as a team in their marriage, and she'd always looked after her share. It had been a partnership and they'd both pulled their weight. Well, they were still partners and what Howard couldn't do she would. It was that simple.

◆   ◆   ◆

Nothing was simple any more. Howard was quickly discovering just how difficult it could be to do the smallest things— and how difficult it was when you couldn't. He couldn't even control when he went to the bathroom, let alone choose the venue. Even Sheba and Humphrey required less upkeep! Thank God for Dana, who took care of him like a pro. And he'd think, *isn't it funny, I can remember changing her diapers*, and then she'd laugh and say, "I was just thinking, Dad, you used to change my diapers." And they'd both smile.

It seemed that when he was wheeled into this hospital, he'd checked his dignity at the door. He didn't feel uncomfortable being tended to by the nursing staff—hell, he'd rather do it himself but somebody had to and they were professionals. And he certainly didn't feel uncomfortable being tended to by his daughter—she was the most professional of them all. Besides, why should he feel more comfort in the hands of a stranger? Her care was a profound expression of her devotion to him, and he felt so lucky to have such an expert nurse. What a kid.

No, Howard didn't mind the professional care of other people—he was just getting extremely bored with not doing it himself. At this point he was basically a barely functioning hunk of flesh with a brain whizzing somewhere inside. He was fed by a tube that required someone else to insert, largely because of the presence of another tube elsewhere that had been inserted to help him breathe. He couldn't shift position in bed when he cramped up or was hot or just tired of being still—someone had to come and turn him, like a rag doll. Yes, things had changed. But Howard looked on the bright side— he wasn't dead and he wasn't in a vegetative state and he was determined not to be this way for long.

Already there were definite changes. They'd reduced the circumference of the trache once, and they'd done so again, presumably to wean him off the tube and start his normal breathing process again. Once the trache was out he knew he'd speak. And eat. Boy, was he sick of that IV. He knew he was getting nourishment, but God, to swallow a big greedy gulp of dinner and then to take another bite and just roll the food around on his tongue, feeling its texture and temperature and the confluence of all the different ingredients merging into the taste that filled his whole mouth, and then swallowing again, and taking another bite for good measure—oh yeah, he missed food a lot.

But he told himself the same thing he thought during physiotherapy, when his mind and body were stressed to the limit: *whatever frustration I endure now will make success that much sweeter*. And then he'd think, *there's going to be a lot of sweetness, because I'm going to have a lot of success.*

◆ ◆ ◆

In the meantime, Howard was occupied by his visitors who came and went through the door of his hospital room to remind him that they were rooting for him. They would pass through in a steady stream, depositing more flowers in the little room. An established roster of regulars was evolving—

one of Kenny Field, Brian Price, Michael Winton, or Jennifer Jackson could always be found reclining by Howard's side, reading him the paper or bringing him up to date on news from the outside world. And of course Helen and his sisters were fixtures, around so much that they'd started blending in with the furniture.

With the fear now mostly gone, the atmosphere was no longer full of tension. The bonding had less urgency, was easier, more relaxed. And the web of family ties kept growing as people whose paths had never really overlapped all that much suddenly spent hours and days together. Food, as always, was a great unifier—there was still a lot of it and they still had to eat, after all. Friendships grow slowly but surely over bagels and sandwiches and cups of coffee.

It had been an interesting journey for Risa. She'd felt obliged to show her face at the hospital, how could she do otherwise? But she felt odd participating in the vigil when she still had so many unresolved issues. It had been difficult, taking such a heavy dose of family all at once. The bat mitzvahs had calmed down of late, though God knows there was still a fairly constant stream of them, and, aside from Passover and the occasional breaking of the fast on Yom Kippur, they really didn't get together all that often. She'd been busy, got married, was happy and focused and *complete* in her life. She hadn't minded the distance so much.

But it was hard to stay distant in this environment. And Risa was confused, because she was starting to forget why she'd want to. This was her family, her roots. Whatever else she did with her life they would always be a part of it, for better or for worse. For better or for worse. She smiled wryly to herself. Like marriage, only you couldn't divorce your family. For better or for worse, in sickness and in health, for richer and for poorer, until death did them part. And she knew all of these people would be fixtures at her side, if God forbid, anything ever happened to her. For better or for worse.

And it wasn't just the family ties that drew her to the hospital more and more, though it was truly nice to be spending so much time together. She was pretty proud of her brother. Howard was so determined, he had such an unbelievable attitude. He'd been so vital and busy, and now he was trapped in this broken body that refused to work. Yet he never seemed to wallow in self-pity, or waver even slightly in his positive outlook. And it was amazing, because every time she'd come to the hospital he'd proudly show off something new he had relearned. And she'd watch him move his left thumb or reposition his leg and she'd share his pride. Unbelievable. Who would have thought? Not her, but she was slowly recognizing that she was being drawn back into Howard and the family. Letting herself be drawn in. Drawing *herself* in. Who would have thought?

The doctors had warned Debbie that Howard might never speak again, but this time she definitely knew they were wrong. She'd heard him speak before the tracheostomy. She knew that he'd prove the doctors wrong. The proof would come when the tube came out.

Dana had cleaned his tracheostomy site, had watched as the nurses removed the tube to suction out all the mucous from the inside. She knew that tube was how he now breathed. It made her nervous. Before it could come out permanently, they had to know whether he'd be able to breathe independently. They'd have to cork the tube to make sure he could breathe on his own. Dana's fear was that her father wouldn't be able to breathe in the middle of the night when no one was around to help. She fell asleep to the strange sound of his breathing, and willed herself to awaken at any change in that sound. It made her feel better.

Howard knew he was ready to become a more functional human being. All signs pointed to his improvement. Physiotherapy was going well, he felt stronger and healthier, although he figured it was pretty easy to feel strong lying in a hospital bed. He could mouth the words, could almost feel them forming in his throat. He was ready.

Finally, the doctors agreed with him. One day one of his nurses, Kim, came in and smiled at him. "Let's get this tracheostomy tube out of you," she said, and capped it. Howard smiled back and mouthed "thank you," knowing that he'd be able to say that aloud pretty soon.

In the meantime, though, his throat had to heal and his breathing had to stabilize. But there were other things he could do while he was waiting for that to happen ... Howard could visualize a heaping, sizzling steak platter from House of Chan, and could feel his sadly neglected mouth start to water. Eating had now moved to the top of his priority list.

Back in the ICU, he had coughed, which they said meant he could probably swallow. One of the nerves affected by stroke is connected to the swallow mechanism, and the gag reflex was impaired. Choking was still a worry, so they had to test that to be certain that swallowing and all the other bodily functions related to eating were working properly. They'd taken him to the testing room—what a relief to have a change of scenery—and given him a barium swallow. Not exactly the first meal he'd had in mind. He'd had to drink down what felt like a gallon of that thick, chalky white goop, which tasted like nothing he'd ever order from House of Chan. Revolting, but necessary. Howard obliged without complaint and swallowed dutifully. It was all in the name of progress.

He was rewarded with liquids. The little white hospital straw that bent toward him became his constant companion as he drank and drank, trying to get his alimentary canal in shape for the real thing. He could hear Debbi and Fidelma in his head: "The more you work the muscle, the stronger it becomes and the greater your control," and he would drink some more.

At last the big day came. Cream of wheat. Howard had never tasted something so incredible in his life. It was like eating the best thing in the world. It was warm, it was thick, and it had *texture*. Howard was in heaven. He took another mouthful and played with it a little, pushing it into every corner of his mouth, through his teeth, under his tongue, squishing up around his gums. Then he scooped it all up with his tongue, sweeping his mouth for remnants and greedily gulping them down. He opened his mouth impatiently for another mouthful, smacking his lips in anticipation and following the spoon hungrily with his eyes until he felt another warm clump on his tongue, and did it all again.

He could eat! He was really on his way to becoming a real person again. The doctors warned him against too much too soon, though—House of Chan would have to wait. Howard knew they were right, considering his tendency to get excited. He knew it would be easy for him to overdo it. That was the story of his life—nothing in moderation. It was a motto he'd cheerfully lived by, and still intended to.

A few more trial runs with cream of wheat and he was ready. His first real meal. He'd never known hospital food could be so delicious. They'd brought him pureed carrots and mashed potatoes and some mushed meat, and the smells were intoxicating. Dana and Kelli were on hand to feed it to him, mainly because just one person spooning and feeding couldn't possibly be fast enough to keep up with his rabid appetite. Dana was so excited that she was practically shoving the mashed potatoes down his throat. This meant so much to her; every little step meant so much! They'd gotten rid of two tubes in the last week. Incredible.

God, this was incredible. He had been right—every moment of frustration and yearning had made this moment of success taste even sweeter.

His mouth had been momentarily distracted, but it didn't take long for Howard to refocus on his primary goal: speaking. He worked at it, trying vainly to push sound out of his mouth. The most he could manage was a weak hiss—his throat had simply not healed enough. As usual, he just had to be patient. As usual, that was difficult for Howard. But he would try, and then when he didn't succeed he'd try to be patient before he tried again. He knew it was only a matter of time. He could wait it out.

In the meantime, he stuck with the chalkboard and the Speak & Spell, and continued to communicate that way. He went to therapy and tried to learn to sit up. He ate his still-delicious hospital food and watched TV and entertained and was entertained by his visitors. Full days, but not a full life.

And then he spoke. At first they weren't sure it wasn't just their imaginations. Howard was in therapy, slumped awkwardly in a sitting position. Dana was straightening him out in her brisk but loving way, taking care of him as usual. And from the corner of his mouth, a sound escaped. "Aaa," he said, and this time they were all certain they had heard it. Debbie, Amie, Dana and Michael Kalles all leaned in, encouraging him to try again. Howard tried again. "Daa," he said, looking at his daughter. Dana felt the tears coming but blinked them back, impatient to hear her father speak. This time he was going to do it.

"Come on, Dad, let's hear you. You can do it," she urged, squeezing his hand tightly.

Slowly, carefully, Howard's mouth formed the sounds of his first word, tasting them carefully before releasing them into the open air of the room.

"Dana," he said.

◆　◆　◆

Rose Ouellet was knitting Howard an afghan. It was starting to get cold now, and winter wasn't far away. It probably got cold in that hospital room. With every stitch of that afghan she thought about and prayed for Howard. It was the least she could do to help.

She called Brian every other day for updates, and Helen on the alternate days. She hadn't yet been back to the hospital. She wanted to give Howard time to recuperate with his family before intruding again. She was so relieved and happy that he hadn't been angry with her, that his whole family had welcomed her as one of them, as one of the many people who loved Howard. But it wasn't her place right now to intrude. She was happy just knowing that he was doing well.

Besides, knitting the afghan made her feel close to him, like she was doing something to help him get well. She hoped he liked it. She knitted a little faster, wanting to finish it for him before winter truly set in.

She was so engrossed that she didn't even hear the phone

ring. Suddenly her husband Roger rushed into the family room where she was knitting, yelling "Get to the phone! Hurry, get to the phone!" Surprised, she looked at him.

She put aside her knitting and stood up. "Who is it?" she asked, but he just laughed as he nudged her over to the phone. It was probably her little niece from out west, but then why was Roger so excited?

Rose was confused. "Hello?"

The voice on the other end was scratchy and hoarse, but unmistakable. "Hi, Rose. Guess who?"

Rose felt a sharp pang of joy. What a wonderful change from when she'd last seen Howard! Now it was she who couldn't talk. She was so overcome with emotion, she could barely respond.

He laughed gleefully, delighted by her delight. "Watch out, Rosie, I got your number now, and I'll be calling all the time."

Rose laughed, thrilled just to hear him speak. "That's just fine with me, Howard. That's just fine with me."

Dr. Shelly Baker was preparing for his day's appointments. A couple fillings, a few cleanings—just an average day at the dentist. He was reviewing charts when the receptionist buzzed.

"Dr. Baker, Dr. Rocket's on the line." Shelly absentmindedly reached for the phone, his eyes still on the chart. *Dr. Rocket's on the line? What the ...* He snatched the receiver. "Hello?"

There was a whisper at the other end. "Hiya, Shelly, I'm back," the voice whispered.

Shelly laughed. "It's good to hear you, Howard."

The whisper turned into a laugh. "It's good to be heard."

◆ ◆ ◆

Howard was having a blast. They'd brought him a cell phone, and he was dialing what seemed to be every person he'd ever known with the wonderful news. God, it was such a kick to surprise them like this! His mother had been overcome, like Rose, and his sisters had laughed with the same delight. He'd called Shawna and Stephen, and he'd been touched by their emotion. Then he'd started on his friends, moving through the Rolodex one by one to personally spread the good news. He'd buzzed every nurse on duty just so he could tell them himself that he was doing fine, and their thrilled and happy reactions fuelled his pride. But they'd taken the phone away because they hadn't wanted him to overdo it, not realizing that they were about five hours too late. Reluctantly he surrendered his new toy and went to sleep, but he was awake and back on the phone at six AM, starting with a slightly dazed Shelly Little and moving methodically down his list.

He was taking a break when his niece walked in for some physiotherapy. God, he was enjoying this!

"Hi, Kelli," he said, enjoying her look of surprise. That was one thing you didn't get with the telephone.

Kelli was beside herself, laughing and smiling and hugging him. "Oh, my God, you can speak! I have to call my mom!"

Howard laughed with her, delighting in the wonder of this new life. "Don't bother," he said. "I already did."

Sweeter. So much sweeter.

Moving

The days passed in a blur of physiotherapy, visitors, and constant little improvements. Now that Howard could talk it really did almost seem like life was back to normal. It was as if a dam in Howard had suddenly burst, releasing pent-up words that gushed forth in a steady stream. From morning until night it seemed like the one constant was Howard's voice, excitedly covering every topic—from what they'd be eating today, tomorrow and next week, to who called and who wrote and who came and who was coming, to how great he felt and how fast he was going to get better and how he'd never felt so *alive*! It was exhausting just being in the room with him, trying to follow the dizzying trains of his thought as they whizzed at warp speed across any and every topic.

It was a relief for Debbie. She'd had to speak for both of them over the past two and a half weeks, had to make phone calls and receive visitors, and explain over and over what had happened and how he was doing, and keep everyone up to date on any changes. Then thank God he'd woken up and the calls and friends had poured in—which was lovely but so tiring, going through the same conversations until she could deliver them flawlessly on autopilot. Now she could relax and let Howard do all the talking. Thank God, she was exhausted.

It was a good thing she didn't want to talk much, because it would have been hard to get a word in edgewise. Howard

loved to talk to everyone, and soon the nurses and his physiotherapists and the doctors and all his visitors were up to date
on how he was feeling and how much he was improving.

"Look at this, Fidelma. See? I can move my hand. Here,
watch, I can do it again. See? There it goes again. Hey, I've been
practising that exercise, and I think I've got it. It's all about
control and discipline, and will power. I want to get better, and
I am. See? Look at my hand. It's getting better, and so am I."

"Hey, Dr. Hu, I am feeling so great. You guys gotta know
that this is the best thing that could have happened to me. The
nurse says my trache's healing faster than she's ever seen. I
believe it, too. It's all in the mind. I don't say, 'why me,' I say,
'why not me'? I was chosen to get sick and I was also chosen
to get better. Did they tell you about what I can do with my leg
now? Here, watch. ..."

"Look, I can sit up by myself! Wait, hold on, I can do this
... there! See? I did it in therapy yesterday and I've been practising. Dana and Amie have been helping me. See? Bet you
never thought I'd come this far, eh, Dr. Lozano? But I did and
I'm going to go further. Did Dr. Willinsky tell you about my
leg? I can bend at the knee a bit now, see ... there! This is so
great, it's just the best thing that's ever happened to me. It's
like being born again. I've been reborn in your hospital. Only
babies can't do all this so fast! Here, watch my hand ..."

Their patient was so funny, the earnest skinny man who
was loudly and happily determined to do everything that the
odds said he couldn't. Dr. Lozano was amused. "I think he
knocked off a few too many neurons," he joked.

At first Debbie also had been amused, but she had begun
to worry a bit. Was this heightened and sustained optimism and
happiness ... normal? The man had almost died, for God's
sake. He couldn't walk, he couldn't function. Wasn't that some-

thing to get a bit *depressed* about, at least sometimes? Not that she *wanted* him to be depressed, she was glad he was so positive and so determined, but at the same time she recognized that this behavior wasn't quite ... Howard. They were lovingly amused by him, but such amusement, however loving it may have been, was not typical of how Howard was usually regarded. Really, who had ever smiled indulgently and said "isn't he cute?" They would *never* have called him cute before. Puppies were cute. Children were cute. Grown men, husbands and fathers, generally were not. Howard definitely was not.

It was another phase about which Debbie would have to educate herself. She asked the doctors about it, hesitant to be anything but optimistic but knowing that optimism without realism would help no one, least of all her husband.

Dr. Lozano was reassuring. "Mrs. Rocket, your husband is on quite a few types of medication, including steroids, which tend to be 'uppers.' Besides which, he has narrowly survived what essentially was the equivalent to a plane crash. It's normal for patients to react emotionally under such circumstances. The technical term for it is 'labile.' For most, emotions run the gamut from euphoria to despondence. It's fortunate for all of you that Dr. Rocket seems to exist only at one end of that spectrum."

So the drugs were a part of it—Howard on uppers. God, he was the last person who would have needed those. She recognized her husband's unfailing optimism as a personality trait, but the force of it still concerned her. She was glad to have her husband back, but he still wasn't quite the one she'd had three weeks ago.

She sighed. This was just another stop on the long road they had to travel. She was just glad to have Howard—glad he was happy and positive and focused on recovery. Sometimes, though, she could use some of his optimism.

◆ ◆ ◆

Howard had never felt so optimistic. This was the greatest challenge that had ever confronted him, everything else was peanuts. And he was winning! He had refused to be pushed down all through this experience, had pushed back harder and inched his way closer to success. It drained him to push so hard, but he knew that was the only way to do anything worthwhile. He was finished going through life halfway.

He pushed hardest in therapy. He was making strong, steady progress; Debbi and Fidelma were impressed. Now that he was able to talk he could give them feedback on how he was feeling and what he was having trouble with. Debbie and Fidelma were glad that he was doing so well, but there were times they thought with longing of those quiet early days in which their patient hadn't been quite so vocal. Silence was a scarce commodity now.

If Howard wasn't talking to them about his therapy or whatever else was on his mind, he was shouting encouragement to the other patients using the gym. He identified with those other people struggling against their bodies. He'd note their progress over the sessions, often asking Debbi and Fidelma about it ("How's the screamer?" or "Did the old guy manage all right with that walker?"). It wasn't enough for Howard to be motivated himself; he had lots of motivation to spare, why not spread it around a little?

"Come on, you can do it!"

"It's for your own good!"

"Don't give up now! Only you can make yourself better!"

Debbi and Fidelma were constantly amazed by their patient. Here he was, himself lying prostrate on a table, capable of such limited movement, focusing on the troubles and triumphs of total strangers. It was impressive that he was capable of such inspiration when he himself was functioning at such a modest level.

It was, however, a level that was rising, bit by bit. Initially his left arm and leg weren't moving at all, but through perseverance and practice Howard was slowly widening their scope of capabilities. He wasn't afraid of trying something impossible, knowing that not being able to do something meant not being able to do it right now. He was patient, he could wait. He knew the payoff of trying everything—even with his odds, something was bound to work. Why not keep trying? Soon he'd run out of things to try. By then, everything would work.

With each new phase of Howard's recovery there developed new routines. Dana still slept by his side, still woke with him in the morning and cared for him as needed, which thank God was less and less every day. Howard's visitors slowly began returning to their normal lives, finding regular spots in their routines to see him until an unofficial visitor's timetable evolved. Howard's days were still full, and now that he could speak he could request movies and TV shows and make phone calls and generally hold court. His room started to take on the personality of a permanent residence, looking less like a florist's shop than a temporary lodging for a very busy and active person. Murray Belzberg had started a trend by bringing him an original gift—a troll. The ugly little toy was strangely cute, standing guard by Howard's bed in a Tarzan suit with a friendly, goofy grin permanently in place. For some reason Howard loved it, and soon it was joined by trolls of all different stripes as the fad caught on

and visitors started bearing trolls over and over again. Soon
Howard amassed an impressive collection.

Now that Howard could eat, he wanted to eat all the time,
and as the requests for new delicacies came pouring out the
food came pouring in. Howard's mealtimes were spent with his
family, and his friends would take turns joining them. He could
feed himself now, using his right hand and trying to use his left.
In the beginning, when he couldn't feed himself, Sonny Prashker
and Michael Wuls had fed him, alternating evenings. Howard
seemed to take the food better that way, gratefully looking forward to the moment when two of his favorite men would enter
his room along with a tray of easy-to-digest hospital food. As
soon as Howard saw them, he would open his mouth like a baby
bird, communicating his excitement for mealtime. It was a
uniquely dependent relationship, yet neither Sonny nor Michael
felt awkwardness in giving, nor did Howard feel shame in re-
ceiving.

Before long Howard was feeding himself, and soon was
able to stomach regular food. They celebrated in style—with
take out from House of Chan, courtesy of Jennifer Jackson. It
was better than he'd imagined it would be. Howard was in
heaven. Only the ever-watchful gaze of Amie, Dana, and Debbie
kept him from shoveling the whole damn meal into his mouth
at once. The entire group—about fifteen happy, hungry people—
sat around the hospital bed feasting and laughing. The decor
may not have been very chic, but there was no lack of spirit
during that meal.

But even Howard couldn't eat all day. Now he was in full
swing, and like most people pent up in a hospital room, he was
restless. He was awake at sunrise and got bored very easily.
His friends had become accustomed to 6 AM phone calls. The
TV was a constant drone in the background, there for him in

case he had no one to play with. That, however, was a rare occurrence. Howard's new-found proficiency on the telephone gave him the freedom to summon and invite. Whenever he thought of something new he wanted to do, novelty and distraction were often just a phone call away. He started getting more involved in business, staying in touch with Jennifer during the day to facilitate his complete re-entry into life. He had Shelly Little set up Amie's laptop nearby, and they had it hooked up to the internet. Howard's voracious appetite for living and experiencing was hard to satisfy, and as a result his room buzzed with activity from morning until night with scarcely a break.

Dr. Lozano was on the fifth floor seeing another patient when his ear was momentarily caught by laughter and noise from down the hall. He knew what his patient was like, but even so knowing was shocked by what he saw. Howard was sitting up in bed with the phone in his hand, talking loudly, while idly channel surfing with the remote in the other hand. He put the person on the other line on hold for a moment to say goodbye to a visitor. Another visitor was already making himself comfortable by the trolls. A computer hummed on the meal tray. The TV droned in the background, quite a bit louder. Howard was telling the person on the other end of the line to fax him. He hung up. The phone rang again. Howard picked it up enthusiastically as his visitor chatted with Dana and the studio audience on TV laughed.

Dr. Lozano was no longer amused. Enough was enough, and this was more than enough. Howard had been on the phone literally all day, in between visitors and usually during. He was hyperstimulated and hyperactive and just plain hyper. He wasn't sleeping or even stopping. His body was trying to heal, but it needed a little help. This had to stop. Time for moderation. Time for sanity. Time for rest. Dr. Lozano banned the phone, banned the computer, banned the constant stream of visitors, banned the delivery of faxes and the mention of business. He banned everything except rest, which was the best medicine for his patient right now.

Rest? Howard didn't want to rest! He'd just started round two of his *life*, for God's sake. There was no time for rest, he had so much lost time to make up for, time when his body had been ill, and the time before that, when his spirit had been ill in another, more insidious way. Howard was looking at the world and it was like an explosion of color, and everything looked different, only this time it was as if a dull film had been wiped away, leaving his life sparkling and new before his eyes. He was greedy for the vast panorama of this new world that he had so barely gained access to. Reluctantly, he accepted that he couldn't leave his body behind. He was disappointed, but he trusted Dr. Lozano and knew that he just wanted what was best for him. Howard was touched at Dr. Lozano's exasperation. He'd let go of clinical detachment for a moment, and in that moment Howard felt that Dr. Lozano cared about him, cared not only that an operation had been successful and a patient was alive, but that a man was living. Howard was glad that his doctors seemed to give a damn. He hoped that his success helped make their own jobs easier. He yawned. Suddenly he was tired.

Missy Mandel had only really known her uncle for a little while. Shawna had always had a special relationship with him— he'd started her in business, and they had that in common, but she herself had never been close with her uncle. He'd always been a fixture in their lives when they were kids—he'd been her dentist, the grownup who took away her candy and stuck scary metal objects in her mouth. Eventually he'd stopped being her dentist and gone back to just being her uncle, her mom's brother and a regular at family functions. She was a kid growing up and that was just how it was. Then she'd had kids herself, and the relationship had changed. Howard adored his great-nieces and lavished attention on them, which made her feel good. They'd go up to his cottage in the summer and play in the lake and the sand, and Missy's kids would bridge the generation between uncle and niece. It was the first time they'd really interacted as adults, and it was an easy and friendly relationship.

Of course Howard had always had a soft spot for Shawna's son, Spencer, but she could understand that, she really could. A chromosomal fluke had made Spencer the first Rocket male in half a century ("*almost* half, *almost*!" Howard used to joke; God forbid that he be mistaken for a fifty-year-old), and it was natural that her uncle would be excited by that. But her uncle loved Kailee and Shai, and that was enough for her. He thought her kids were special too. Well, so did she.

The children had been too upset to visit Howard at first. Missy tried going with Kailee once—she thought he'd like that—but Kailee had been terrified just walking into the hospital. The dull yellow light, the windowless halls, the stretchers and tubes and sick people reaching out toward the sweetness and health of a two-year-old. There was no way she'd stand one look at her pasty gray uncle with the mean-looking bruises under his eyes. They were kids—this wasn't their laughing, loving uncle.

But now Howard was on the upswing, and he looked like a person again. The girls would recognize their Uncle Howie. Missy started taking them to visit, and each time they'd bring him a present. She loved painting and drawing with her children, and felt pride in seeing the walls of Howard's rooms covered with their handiwork. Every day the girls would ask how Uncle Howie was, and could Mommy take them to see Uncle Howie again? Mommy was happy to. Did Mommy think Uncle Howie wanted a toy? Did Mommy think Uncle Howie wanted a picture? Mommy thought so. Did Mommy think Uncle Howie wanted a book? Mommy thought for a moment and smiled. Mommy thought that was a great idea.

She knew the perfect book. A book about wishing. A book about family. A book about trying really really hard, and succeeding. It was called *The Magic Pebble* and it was one of their favorites. She bundled the kids into the car and together they started the now-familiar trip to the hospital. Missy was excited—she knew her uncle would appreciate the theme and message of the book. She wanted to give him something that could help him stay positive.

On impulse, she pulled over and stopped the car.

"Come on, girls, we have to find the magic pebble for Uncle Howie." Rooting around in the dirt by the side of the road suddenly seemed like a great idea. Together they examined local rock specimens for size and shape. The chosen pebble had to have magic in it. For some reason Missy didn't doubt that such a pebble existed. She felt like a kid herself.

"Here it is!" yelled Shai, offering a small rock to her mother for appraisal. Missy examined it. It was small, smooth, and round. Just what a pebble should be. Exhilarated by success, they clambered back into the car and headed to the nearest paint store to touch up nature's handiwork. A few sprays and the pebble glistened. Now they were ready to visit Uncle Howie.

As they rode up in the elevator to see him, Missy realized that there might be other visitors with him—Howard was seldom alone, and certainly not so on a weekend. She was oddly disappointed by that. She didn't think this sort of magic worked with other grown-ups around.

But when they got to Howard's room, it was quiet. He was sleeping, which probably meant a coffee break for who-ever had been with him, most likely Debbie or one of the girls. Missy looked at her uncle lying there, a prisoner in that bed, and hoped that there was some magic somewhere that could help him. It didn't have to be from the pebble.

She wasn't sure if she should let him sleep, but he must have just been dozing because suddenly his eyes were open and he was smiling and holding his good arm out to the girls. Missy felt the same rush of pleasure she always did when anyone reached out to her kids. She was happy to share them. She held them up to his face so they could give him their little kisses, and then she kissed him herself. Time for some magic.

Missy loved reading to her kids, or to her class at school. It was wonderful to build and follow a story with children, who ate up every detail with excitement and wonder. But she'd never read aloud in front of another adult. Not even at seders when they'd go around the table taking turns reading from the Haggadah, not even out loud from a newspaper to her husband over breakfast. The sound of her own voice had always seemed stiff and strange in that context, and she'd always been too self-conscious to overlook it. This would be the first time. She wondered why she wasn't nervous. After all, her uncle had been a grown-up for her whole life. Perhaps it was because she could see something of Howard's excitement at his progress in her kids, who daily learned some wonderful new secret about how to interact with the world. It was like he was a kid again, starting from scratch, having to learn to do everything again for the first time. And there were so many firsts to come.

Well, this was a first for her.

"Uncle Howie, this book is called *The Magic Pebble*. It's about someone who suddenly changes, and tries really really hard to return to his family as his old self, and how he finally does." Her uncle was smiling, but she could see emotion in his face. "We know that you can do the same thing, and to help you along we brought you your very own magic pebble." She motioned to Shai, who shyly placed her little hand over her uncle's big one, dropping the pebble in his open palm. His hand closed over it into a fist, tightly.

That was her cue. "Once upon a time ..." The words just came, as if Howard were one of her own children. The three of them were sitting at rapt attention, listening to her voice as she animated the pictures. She felt great! There was a connection, a closeness right now in this room, a current flowing through them that was powered by her words. And her uncle, who had once read to her, was listening solemnly, letting each word fall slowly on his ears so he could savor the message and the meaning.

I wish I could go home, oh I wish I could go home ...

They sat like that for a while in the still, small room with the fingerpaintings on the wall and the trolls by the bedside, as the cadence of Missy's voice gently filled their ears. The two girls snuggled warmly into their uncle, who held them as all the while his good hand still clutched a small, painted rock.

It was time to ascend another level. Phone calls and videos and computer games were diversions, but they didn't divert for long. It was time for more. He couldn't move himself, but he could sit up now and maintain some degree of control.

He wanted out of his hospital room, at least for a moment or two. Was it too much to ask?

No, sighed Dr. Lozano, splintering under the sustained onslaught of Howard's pleas. It wasn't too much to ask. Dr. Rocket would be transferred to a wheelchair and taken on a little stroll. Yes, weather permitting he could be taken outside. It was winter, after all, and did he need to remind his patient that three weeks ago he'd almost died?

Precisely. Howard knew how long it had been. He'd watched the sun rise every day outside his room, strained to catch a stray breeze through the narrow hospital window. It had been three weeks since he'd been outside. No wonder he was pale and pasty.

A nurse came with them for the trip, just in case. Dana pushed and Debbie and Amie walked alongside, feeling Howard's excitement growing along with their own. For them, these halls had gained weary familiarity. For Howard, they were as exciting as cream of wheat had been—now was the time for the ordinary and the humdrum to be invested with the bright shiny newness of the unexperienced. He loved the fact that people were bustling to and fro, and he gave a loud, happy greeting to everyone he saw, shouting *hello!* through open doors and down busy hallways. As they rolled through the crowded lobby, Howard laughed aloud. Life! Vitality! This was what it was all about. People living, doing their own thing, interacting and making their lives and the world go forward every day. He was so very, very glad to be a part of it again.

They were nearing the doors, seeing them slide open and close automatically, letting in natural daylight and then closing firmly against it as people came and went. Then the doors opened for him—it seemed that they'd opened just for him—and he was outside.

It all hit him at once, a physical wave over the senses with an emotional wave in tow. Howard felt the sharp cold of the air against his face even as he tasted its sweetness, and the brightness struck his whole body as if he had eyes everywhere reeling from the brilliance of it all. Then his eyes and body slowly adjusted to the light, and he stopped feeling and looked around at the world he'd left three weeks ago and had almost left for good.

There on his right was the Bathurst Street traffic he'd been listening to from five storeys above. It was wonderful to watch the cars streaming by in brief flashes of color, honking and speeding and weaving and starting and stopping. Life going on right under his window. He looked up at the side of the hospital with its banks of identical windows looking out, and knew that behind every window was a person who would feel this way when they got out. If they got out. Howard closed his eyes for a moment and was thankful for this and every other blessing of his new life.

Someone was speaking. Howard was dimly aware of the nurse, asking if he wanted to go back inside. But he wasn't really listening. After three long weeks he had sunshine on his face.

Walking

Left foot, right foot. Left foot, right foot. It was so easy, made so much sense. In his head he was doing it, without even thinking about it. So why the hell was nothing happening? He gripped the bar. Left foot, right foot. He looked down. Nothing. Damn!

He could stand now, if he held on to something and got his balance just right. His right arm was aching from the compensation, but he tried not to notice. He had to concentrate on moving that damn leg. He could feel a hand on his chest, steadying him. His physiotherapist, sensing weakness. He wished he could walk away from that hand, but he needed it. Damn!

"Take it easy, Howard, it's not going to happen all at once." His physiotherapist again. He hadn't even realized that he'd spoken aloud. All attention had been on his leg.

His physiotherapist was gently guiding him back to his wheelchair. "That's enough for today, anyhow. Keep doing your exercises and we'll pick up again tomorrow," she said, supporting him from behind as he eased himself down into a sitting position. Back in the familiar wheelchair. At least he could move around now. At least he had a world past his hospital bed.

He was in a whole new world now, a whole new stage in his new life. He'd been transferred from the Toronto Hospital to The Queen Elizabeth Hospital (now known as Toronto Rehabilitation Institute after a series of amalgamations with other health care institutions). A huge step. It had taken all of one month to have a stroke, almost die, fight to survive, learn to breathe, eat, talk, and move by himself, and find his life again. It had been a busy month.

Now he was at the Toronto Rehabilitation Institute (TRI), and he was serious about getting better. Dr. Lozano had sent Howard off with his blessing, finally convinced that his patient's miraculous recovery was for real. Howard had bid goodbye to Debbi and Fidelma, promising to make them proud, knowing that he was already halfway there. It wasn't every day that they got to see their patients meet with such success, but then again Howard was no ordinary patient.

He'd been ready to leave the Toronto Hospital. He was more than stable; his body was strong again, ready to work hard to recuperate and relearn. He had been glad to bid fare-well to his hospital room overlooking Bathurst Street, had gladly said goodbye to the four walls that had been all he could see in any direction for far too long. It was the sense of captivity that had frustrated him the most, laying helpless in a bed with bars on both sides, tethered by an IV or an oxygen mask, locked into position by his inability to move. Even when he'd started getting better he hadn't been free; he'd still been trapped in that hospital bed, chafing against his dependency.

He'd tasted freedom a couple of times, though, and it had been so very sweet. The sweetest was the first time, about two weeks into his convalescence. He'd been bedridden for a good long while, gone through his share of sweats, accumulated his share of grime. It had been two weeks and Howard had been ready for some cleansing. Dana had done what she could with dampened facecloths and towels, but Howard had simply not been well enough to move. Thankfully, wonderfully, that had eventually changed, and he'd been given clearance to be moved those few all-important feet to the washroom, with the promise of its shower.

He almost hadn't noticed the nurse propping him up. Even if he could have moved he would have just stood there under the falling water, letting it splash over him and wash away the heaviness of the past two weeks. The water was mild, but it cooled and refreshed and warmed and invigorated him all at the same time. He turned his face into the stream, squeezing his eyes joyfully against its pressure, then bending his head so that the water could carve its way through his hair and run down his neck and over his back. He opened his mouth and let it spray across his tongue, swallowing some and then spitting it out like a kid. And all the while, the water kept running and he kept on thriving on its freshness, thinking *this is what freedom feels like, it's this simple and it's this pure.* He had never known that about a shower before. How lucky he was to know that now.

Freedom came more easily now, with the wheelchair. Suddenly Howard was mobile again and he absolutely loved it. He had one good arm, which was enough to roll himself all over the hospital, sometimes outside if it wasn't too cold. They'd taught him how to move himself from the bed to the chair, and now he had the motion down pat. It hadn't taken him long. Now, when his family and friends came to visit, he rolled himself out to greet them, at the elevator or in the hallway or in the lobby. They never pushed him.

Dana was now one of those visitors. Her tenure as roommate had ended with his stay at the Western; the TRI would allow no such accommodation. At first Dana had balked at leaving her dad alone after three solid weeks of constant togetherness—the instinct to protect and care for him was difficult for her to ignore. But they both recognized that her Dad was in a new phase now, becoming more able to care for himself. He had needed her at the Western—though, in truth, she wondered if really she hadn't needed him more—but now the worst was over and the healing had more than begun. It was right that a semblance of normal life should resume, right for both of them. Dana had already missed almost a month of school, had simply turned her back on her studies and education without a second thought. She had her priorities straight. But Howard didn't want her to give up any more for him, and no longer needed her to. He'd learned to accept her growing up and moving on for twenty-one years—funny, now it was time for her to do the same.

Amie, too, had something she needed to do. She had up and left her program in its final stages, and the thought of completing her MBA had not even entered her mind while her father was in danger. She hadn't even cared. But time was passing quickly, and her program would be drawing to a close in time for the Christmas holidays. With or without her. Now that her dad was all right, thank God, she suddenly realized that she was weeks away from graduating, and that might be in jeopardy. Everyone was in agreement: if she could salvage her degree at this point, she should return to Tokyo and do it. No one was more adamant about this than her father—he couldn't think of a better business partner.

It was funny, thought Amie, how other priorities suddenly came to the fore when everything else was working out. She felt guilty for being greedy. At first she'd just begged God to let him live, please just let him live. When he was out of the woods she had started praying for his recovery—first the big things, and then all the other details. Now that she'd been so very lucky and had all of these wishes granted, she found herself offering up a prayer that all the other things would work out. How unimportant these details had seemed three weeks ago, how selfish she felt for caring about them now. But life had to go on, and she wanted everyone, including herself, to be as happy in that life as was possible. It was okay for life to go on. It was right that it should. She booked her ticket.

So they would come to the TRI, Debbie and Amie and Dana and the two Michaels, and the family parties would resume a few streets over in downtown Toronto. Now that the urgency had subsided, the gatherings had become more relaxed, and friends came less often but stayed longer. It was a different sort of pace but it suited them all, adding a dimension of intimacy borne of close contact instead of close quarters. There were worse ways for families and friends to get to know each other. They'd already been through one of them.

Howard was progressing rapidly and everyone was impressed. His family and friends kept marveling at his energy, his attitude, his drive. Howard was happy to take some of the credit, but he knew that a good part of it did not belong to him. He had Glenda to thank for it.

Glenda was his nurse. That was her official title, anyway. In reality, she was his coach, tough and gruff on the outside but pulling for him all the way, bringing out the fighter in him, refusing to indulge or coddle, demanding nothing short of one hundred percent. He'd arrived at the Toronto Rehabilitation Institute his usual hyperactive self, excited and unrestrained and used to being the center of a whole lot of people's attention. Glenda and the other caregivers had been briefed on this new patient, knew that there was extensive family involvement in his care and that oversight of his treatment was likely. She had thought she was ready for his arrival. Not quite.

The first thing that struck her was his youth. The elevator doors opened and out rolled an earnest-looking fellow, all smiles, with a cap on his head, talking a hundred miles an hour. It caught her a bit off guard, which allowed Howard to get in the first word. Howard had been assigned to one of her rooms—524—and as she walked her patient and his wife to his new room, Howard continued to prattle on about how excited he was to be there and how quickly he was going to get better and how great he felt. Glenda didn't mind; she wanted her patients to feel comfortable under her care. Often they were nervous, and rambling on seemed to calm them. They usually ran out of steam after a while.

This one had a lot of steam, apparently. Glenda realized with both amusement and annoyance that she wasn't getting a word in edgewise. Who was this man? She was trying to tell him important information, and he wasn't having any of it. He was busy talking about his life, his stroke, his work, his daughters, and how his life had changed. When he wasn't speaking, his wife was asking questions. How many hours per day of physio? What other therapies would he be undergoing? Would he be on the same schedule of medication? How long before he was ready to come home? Glenda's head was spinning. She really had not been ready for this.

At the end of their three-hour session, Glenda knew about Japan and Tridont and seeing the light and Spencer and the ICU and the Michaels and close to everything else. She hadn't officially admitted Howard because she hadn't quite been presented with an opportunity to speak. This was not going as planned. An unconventional approach was required.

Glenda decided to allow her patient some time to get used to his new surroundings, time to calm down and get over the initial excitement of arrival. She wanted to speak to him when he was focused, and when he was alone. They had a great deal of work to do.

She walked into his room and he opened his mouth. Glenda wasn't about to make the same mistake twice. She knew what she was doing. She was holding a shirt, and she tossed it on the bed.

"Put this on. I'll be back in five minutes."

Glenda was gone before Howard had figured out what was going on. He looked at the shirt. A challenge. Well, he was up for that. He reached for it.

When Glenda came back he was still struggling with it. He'd managed to pull it over his left arm, but had only been able to fasten two buttons. He was working hard on the third, but it wouldn't quite catch.

"Brace the left side of the shirt with your left arm. Use your right arm to position it." Howard looked up, then did so. His left arm wouldn't stay. Glenda reached over and steadied it for him, then let go. It stayed. Howard turned back to the button, and manipulated it into place. He looked at Glenda again. He made no move to speak. It was her turn.

"You're here for a reason, and so am I. We have to work together on this, and in order to do so I need some information. What's your plan? What do you want me to do for you? What do you want to do for you?"

Howard was taken aback, but he knew those answers. "I want to walk. I want to drive. I want to work. I want to be able to do everything."

"You won't be able to do everything. Nobody can. But you can set goals and achieve them. What else?"

"I want people to learn from me, I want to teach them about my stroke, to warn them. This thing happened to me, maybe for a reason, maybe not. But I can't go back to being ignorant and I don't think I can let anyone else be ignorant if I can help it."

"Okay, good. We have goals, we have a purpose, we have a plan. I think we can work together." Howard opened his mouth to speak again, and she cut him off. She wasn't finished. "But—you have to listen to and accept my goals, too. My goals are what I need from you; you have to help me before I can help you. I need you to give me at least fifteen minutes a day, no matter how exhausted you may be from therapy or who's coming to visit. Agreed?" Howard nodded.

"I need you to follow my instructions, and to listen to me. Listening is hard work, Howard, and my guess is that you're used to being listened to. Listening requires patience, and it's tough to be patient from where you're at. I know that. But it doesn't mean I'll accept it as an excuse. Agreed?" Howard nodded again.

"You're going to fall on your head and that's okay, because it's the only way you'll listen and it's the only way you'll learn. I won't let you fall too hard."

Howard had thought he was working hard, but he worked harder for Glenda than he would have thought possible. He still threw himself into phsyio and occupational and speech therapy, but there was a difference now; he *thought* about what he was doing and how he was doing it. He began realizing that it wasn't just how hard you pushed, but *how* you pushed that really made the difference. That was something Glenda had taught him.

Howard responded well to Glenda's "tough love." He enjoyed rising to the challenge of her expectations and demands, felt proud when he saw that he'd pleased her, craved her approval. Glenda did not lavish praise on her patients unless it was truly deserved, and Howard knew that approval from Glenda was hard won and well earned. He tried very hard to earn it.

Glenda recognized something special in Howard, and really felt strongly about helping him to get better. It was more than the professional desire to see a patient get well; she wanted to see *this* patient get well. In spite of the gruffness that her position required, she was really becoming quite attached to Howard, whose exuberance and excitement and enthusiasm were refreshing and endearing. He was like an excitable puppy whose tail was in perpetual wagging mode.

She was more than a nurse to him, anyhow. When she had pledged to work with him to help him reach his goals and resume his life, she had undertaken more than fifteen minutes a day. For the first time, Howard didn't feel like he had to offer support. With his family and friends he tried to stay "up" because he felt they needed assurance from him that he was going to be all right. It was assurance he was happy to give, but it was draining. He was more emotional than he'd ever been, and had become accustomed to a good cry now and then. His family was accepting and comforting of this new emotional streak, but it worried them, he could tell. The Howie Rocket they knew never cried, was always pumped, excited, and on top of the world, even from the confines of a hospital bed. So he tried to be encouraging, and most of the time it didn't take any effort. Like at the Western, he would shout his encouragement across gyms and hallways and cafeterias, wheeling around to different patients with whom he now shared a unique bond, trying to infuse them with a little of his optimism. Yet there were times when the sheer exhaustion of it all did get to him, when the weight of trying to move a foot or a finger was crushing upon him, and when he felt like he needed to just let go. Glenda tried to be there for him in those times, taking her own lunch break to visit him in his room, giving up her own free time to be there for him. Somehow, it wasn't a sacrifice. Theirs was a partnership that worked.

◆ ◆ ◆

He was used to his routine: physiotherapy, occupational therapy, speech therapy, Glenda, exercises, visitors, meals, and quite a bit of medication. The line-up of drugs was really quite impressive: decadron, dilantin, coumadin, colace for stool softening, zantac for heartburn, heparin to thin his blood. One couldn't be too careful. Howard was just glad that he was no longer getting his medication through tubes. What a joy to be able to pop a pill. He felt great, so someone must have been doing something right.

Feeling great meant feeling restless. That was where the wheelchair came in. The chair changed everything, really. He could go anywhere now, although the hospital was reluctant to set him loose on Toronto; in his short stay, they'd begun to realize that Howard didn't like to acknowledge any limits. But at Glenda's urging they had let him go out for dinner one night with his family, for Chinese food at Lichee Garden around the corner.

He'd felt like a real person again, almost indistinguishable from all the other diners. Like him, everyone was sitting down. Like him, everyone was hungry. It was true that using a knife and fork was a bit of a problem, and damned if he'd be able to use chopsticks. But he had one good hand and one healthy appetite, and that was pretty much all he needed. He'd let Michael Kalles push the wheelchair on the way over because he'd wanted to save his energy for the meal, and now he was glad he had. He wanted to savor this sense of being in the real world, to experience the full height of belonging.

For the first time, Debbie was realizing what that belonging required. It was one thing for Howard to be sitting happily stuffing himself at the table—it was quite another to actually get him there. Debbie had never really noticed whether buildings had ramps or stairs or elevators, had never bothered to look at whether curbs were flattened for access or whether sidewalks were smoothly paved. All of these things made a difference to someone in a wheelchair. Debbie had never thought about how these things might affect other people because they'd never affected her. Now there were buttons to push and special entrances, special elevators and facilities and passes. It was very new to her. She sighed. She was getting used to everything being new to her.

Howard was progressing extraordinarily well, and the hospital had promised that soon he'd be able to go home on weekends. Debbie had quickly realized that there was much to be done in anticipation of his arrival. Their front door could be reached only by high brick steps with no railing, leading off a cobblestone walkway. Their bedroom was upstairs; all that was on the first floor was the kitchen, bathroom and living room. No shower, no bed. In short, no access. That had to be changed.

Michael Kalles knew a contractor, and within a few days, it was. A new ramp led from the driveway to the front door. A metal bar was installed in the bathroom along the wall. They special-ordered a hospital bed for the living room, and reorganized the room to accommodate a patient. The kitchen table was raised slightly so that a wheelchair could fit. And Howard's favorite snacks were placed on the lower shelves in cupboards and the refrigerator so he wouldn't have to be dependent on his family for everything he wanted. Taped to the fridge was a chart outlining when Howard received his various medications. Debbie took a look around her new house. The transformation was complete, they hadn't forgotten anything. Welcome home, Howard.

Welcome home, indeed. Howard couldn't believe what he felt when he wheeled through the front door. So familiar, yet everything had changed. He was looking at everything from a new vantage point now, and the physical perspective had shifted. The stairs seemed to stretch upward far higher than he'd ever noticed, and his usual habit of taking them two at a time seemed incomprehensible. There were no more usual habits. His house had to be relearned.

He wheeled around in the kitchen. He'd never noticed what an obstacle that island in the middle was. And there was no way he'd be reaching the sink. The table had been raised but it felt strange, and the view from his kitchen window seemed to have shifted. He couldn't tell if something was really different or if the shift was inside him. He wheeled to the fridge and looked inside. Anything he would want was on the lower shelves. Trust Debbie to look after him. He'd already noticed the fresh flowers.

Debbie was calling him to the living room. His room. He went to wheel through the adjoining door through the kitchen, but couldn't fit the chair between the wall, the dining room table and the sideboard. So damn much to get used to. He pivoted and went out the way he came in, emerging in the vestibule and wheeling himself down the hall. Debbie was standing by the bed, smiling at him. The hospital blue looked absurdly out of place among the rich mahogany and subtle earth tones of their living room; their decorator would *not* be pleased. But Howard was. It wasn't his bed, but it was in his home, and that was good enough, at least for right now. It was just too bad that he couldn't share it with his wife. Time enough for that, he smiled to himself. He wasn't ruling anything out.

Debbie was smiling back. It was good to be home.

Home was for weekends, and they were over too quickly. It was incredible to be in his own place, despite being confined to the ground floor. For the first time his family weren't visitors, and being with him didn't have to mean being perched on the side of his bed or on one of those orange plastic chairs that hospitals seemed to buy in bulk. It was nice just being around everyone doing everyday things. He'd so missed everyday things. He loved hearing the key turn in the lock, hearing Dana yelling down to him from upstairs, hearing the phone ring and the toilet flush and the microwave beep. The everyday sounds of life going on. Incredible.

They'd set him up pretty comfortably in the living room, with a TV and a VCR and the stereo and the phone. Next to him the coffee table was littered with books, snacks, pills, and remote controls. All the essentials. He couldn't read yet, his vision was nowhere near ready for that, even with his glasses, but he loved being read to. It was peaceful, and nice. He didn't really pay much attention to content, it was the warmth of a soothing and familiar voice that he loved.

Comfortable as he was, there were difficulties. Howard was still a recovering patient with significant requirements, and his family was simply not equipped to provide full-time nursing care. He needed more help than they could give him. He still had difficulty going to the bathroom by himself, and needed help transferring from the wheelchair to the toilet. And although he'd mastered the various remote controls, he still couldn't change a CD or a videocassette by himself. There were many things he could do with one hand, but there were many, many more that required two.

Wonderful as it was to be home, there was simply not much for him to do on the main floor of his medium-sized home. If it hadn't been December, he might have been able to wheel around his neighborhood, but snow, ice, and slush weren't exactly a wheelchair's best friends. He loved his family, but he simply wasn't ready to be home yet. If he was honest, he would admit to himself that he was bored. He missed the long stretches of hallway in the Toronto Rehabilitation Institute, missed the attention and ambition of therapy, missed Glenda's visits and the confidence they gave him, missed visiting other patients to deliver his daily dose of optimism. Soon, home would be right. All in good time.

And he was working very hard to get to that time quickly. Therapy was going well, because finally his body seemed to be listening, kind of. Left foot, right foot. Left foot, right foot. He'd look down, and for the first time he was starting to see a response. It was taking every ounce of energy he had, but he was learning to drag his left foot forward and make it accept some of his weight. It was a slow, draining process that required steadying bars and hands, but he was doing it, and that was progress. The possibility of not walking again had never entered his mind. He would do it.

He remembered Amie and Dana as babies learning to walk. Crawling was the first taste of freedom and independence, and he could still recall the determination and joy of his daughters as they hauled their clumsy bodies along the floor to examine and explore their world. But what stood out in his mind the most was the memory of how they looked standing for the first time. Their little arms had to work a bit before they were strong enough to pull the rest of them up, and they had to struggle to get arms and legs and back to work together. It had been marvelous to watch them try, to see them fail and think and then try something a little different. And when they had finally failed enough, it had been the most amazing thing to see them pulling themselves all the way up, wobbly and unsure at first but then surprisingly steady, balancing against the side of the crib as they stood upright for the first time. Their view from the crib had altered forever, and so had they.

Howard now understood what his daughters had felt at that time. He labored to wring some use out of his latent left limbs, had to relearn the patterns of their movement and their relation to the rest of his body. He had to find the balance between relying on his good side and forcing himself to use his bad side. It wasn't easy. Like his infant daughters, he tried and tried and tried, and kept on failing. But each time he learned what not to do, and tried something a little different. Maybe this time it would work.

It almost did, many times. But he still wasn't strong enough, he needed help, constantly, and the wheelchair was always waiting in the wings. His physiotherapist assured him that his progress was excellent, amazing really, but Howard was getting frustrated. December was slipping away and constant convalescence was wearing a bit thin. He'd always known it was going to take time, but he was getting impatient, dammit! The curve was flattening, and it scared him. He didn't want to stop improving, not when he still had so far to go.

He couldn't believe how the time had flown. Amie and Dana were back at school, visits were slowly transforming into phone calls, and family get-togethers were now planned instead of the natural by product of daily activity. Life was going on, and that was okay. Actually, it was great. He just wanted to go with it, all the way.

The family would be getting together soon, actually. At Marsha's for New Year's Day brunch. He was excited, he was going to wear his tuxedo. Looking like an able-bodied person for a change had definite appeal. Come to think of it, this would be the first official family get-together since his stroke: the first event on his post-stroke social calendar. Sure, he'd made it out of the hospital for dinner a few times and entertained people at his house on weekends, but this was different. This was going out in a tux. If nothing else, Howard loved going out in a tux.

They had decided to have the party during the day so that all the kids could come. Howard got himself ready in the downstairs bathroom, almost getting his tuxedo on without help. There was no way he could manage cufflinks, though. Couldn't get too ambitious. He had shaved, loving the scent of the aftershave. It was the smell of a guy who had somewhere to go. He smoothed some gel through his hair, clean and neat thanks to his barber, Gino, from Capucci Hair Studios. Gino had taken the subway to the hospital in order to give Howard a haircut at 7:30 AM, before his own salon opened. It had been a nice thing to do, not to mention a pretty decent haircut.

The dogs were going crazy. That had to mean that Dana and Michael were here to pick them up. Howard took a last look in the mirror. His tux hung loosely around his body—having a stroke clearly didn't do wonders for one's physique—and his skin was a little on the pale side. But, all things considered, he looked pretty good. He smiled, and his reflection smiled back, revealing a set of teeth that were a credit to his profession. He was ready to go. Happy New Year.

There were cars parked all along the street, but the driveway was clear. Life went on, but his family remembered. They pulled up to the front of the house, and the door opened wide. Even though the mid-winter temperatures were frigid, Marsha and Shelly Baker were already outside, greeting their guest of honor. Shawna and Stephen were at the front door with their kids, and Spencer was pointing to the car. Howard couldn't wait to hold those kids on his lap. He could see other family members filling the doorway, and he was filled with the urge to run. But the wheelchair behind him was a reminder that he'd have to wait for that. He felt a sudden surge of resentment. That chair had been a ticket to freedom, but now it was as much of a prison as the four walls of his hospital room had been. He couldn't deal with that today.

"I want to walk in." He heard his own voice and realized he'd said it aloud. Committed to it. Debbie already had the chair positioned for his transfer. She looked at him, and he shook his head. "No," he said. "I don't even want to bring the chair in the house. I can do it."

Debbie looked worried, but she pulled the chair away from the open car door. Dana was outside, ready to help her father to the ground. She motioned Shelly over to Howard's other side.

Howard could feel his heart pounding. His senses were alive in the sub-zero January chill. He was going to do this. With Dana and Shelly each supporting an arm, he swung his legs around so his feet were touching the ground. Putting all his weight on his right leg and bracing himself with his right arm, he stood. He was so close to that doorway, but right now it seemed a great distance to travel. Slowly, he tested his left leg, transferring some of his weight. This was the test. His leg was weak, but he'd been working hard. He felt the pressure and the strain, but he felt his muscles responding. On his left, Shelly was holding him up, but so was his leg. Now the test.

Like his infant daughters over two decades ago, he'd had to learn how to use all the parts of his body together. Now he braced himself with his arms, using and applying every muscle from shoulder to fingertip. His hand was spread wide against Shelly's chest for leverage, slung over Dana's shoulder for balance. In order to take a step, his left leg would have to support the movement of his right. Tensing his body, he tried to remember what it had felt like in the gym at the TRI. Left foot, right foot. Left foot, right foot. Shelly and Dana had him. There was no reason not to just do it.

So he did. Before he even realized what had happened his right foot was in front of him and his left was pulling itself along the ground, and suddenly his body had shifted and his right foot wasn't in front of him anymore. Applause was coming from the open doorway. Suddenly his family seemed a lot closer. Left foot, right foot. Left foot, right foot. It was true, Dana and Shelly were helping him and holding him. But they weren't dragging him, and they weren't carrying him. Somewhere in between, it was coming from him.

Living

A key was turning in the lock, sending the dogs into a frenzy. Their master walked in and threw his keys on the side table, shrugging off his jacket as he walked into the kitchen. The dogs were following him, stampeding his lower legs, demanding attention. He stopped for a moment to give them their due, then continued toward the phone to check messages, sifting through the day's mail while he listened. Saving one message and deleting three, he put the phone down and walked out of the kitchen and started up the stairs. Howard was in a business suit and felt like wearing sweats. A change of clothes was in order.

He climbed stairs now, easily. He walked, sometimes with a cane, sometimes without. He drove his car, and figured that he was actually far safer on the road than he'd ever been. He exercised, logging solid blocks of time on the exercise bike. He rode a real bike, too, with three wheels. He stood, and he sat, and he ate, and he breathed. One year after his stroke, Howard Rocket did it all.

It had been one tough year, but he was back now and planned to stay. He had re-entered life with a vengeance. Come to think of it, he'd more than just re-entered, he'd reformed it, reshaped it, renewed it. His was a life once lost and then found, and when he found it again he'd found something new. New priorities. New challenges. New goals.

Now Howard Rocket saw his life as part of a greater whole, interacting with the world around him in the complex, intertwined oneness of humanity. It wasn't enough for him just to love and make the most of his own life—he now knew that the worth of his own life was to be found in what he did with it.

He remembered sitting in the Toronto Rehabilitation Institute at his first meeting with Glenda, as she challenged him to define what he wanted to achieve. He had said he wanted to teach people, warn them, share with them his knowledge of how valuable life is. He knew he had done that, was doing it every day. Howard had taken his story and shared it, speaking at meetings, gatherings and conferences. He knew his was a remarkable success story, and that people had to know that this world held miracles as well as tragedies, and that either and both could happen to them. He also knew, while he'd been able to get where he was because of his will and determination, that luck had more to do with it than anything else. One year ago, the odds were he would die. He had been strong, but he also had been lucky.

He tried to share that luck with others. Every week, Howard and Dana and Amie would pick up a stack of sandwiches and some soup and distribute them randomly downtown. There were always many grateful recipients. Howard knew this wasn't solving the problems of Toronto's homeless, but it made a difference for a moment, and perhaps for longer. He knew he could just donate money, which he did, but he wanted to make a difference personally, to recall the profound feelings of gratitude he had felt for all his good fortune. He knew from experience how easy it was to take it all for granted.

Howard continued to go back to the Toronto Rehabilitation Institute to visit the other patients, offering encouragement as a living example of recovery. He had spent his few months there working hard and watching others work hard. Their struggles were an inspiration to him in those wheelchair-bound days, and he had strived to be an inspiration in return. He'd been quite a character at the Institute, speeding through the halls in his wheelchair. There were times when he'd put on his rollerblades, just to be mischievous, and tool around in a helmet and gear, letting everyone know that he'd be doing it for real soon enough. He'd loved sensing the floor moving under his wheels, smooth and yielding but with a touch of friction. Friction. He'd come to love it. Friction meant movement and power and resistance overcome. He'd wanted to organize a wheelchair race through the halls, but the hospital didn't jump at his offer. Still, his enthusiasm and support directed to the other patients had been warmly received. It had made everyone's job much easier.

Howard knew he had made a difference in at least one person's life. Stan Cohen was a man about his age who had lived in his neighborhood and they had moved in similar circles over the years. Their kids had both gone to the same school, and knew each other. Yet Stan and Howard had never met; there had never been a reason to. But in November, 1995, almost a month after Howard's stroke, Stan and his wife Susan had been in a car accident on the highway to Kingston. Their car had gone out of control and slammed into the sheer rock face flanking the highway. Stan suffered critical injuries including a broken neck, head trauma, and a crushed right hand. Tragically, Susan had been killed.

Stan retained no memory of that day, nor of the next four weeks spent in critical condition at the hospital. He hadn't even been told what had happened until four and a half weeks later, when he had partially recovered. When he could understand.

Stan hadn't wanted to understand. Hadn't wanted to ac-

knowledge the loss after twenty-nine and a half years of marriage. Hadn't wanted to face the enormity of life without her.
Hadn't wanted to accept that any of it had happened.

But he was still alive, and his body was healing itself. He
was transferred from Sunnybrook Health Science Centre to the
TRI for further recovery. They told him he would walk again.
They told him he would use his hand again. They told him he
would live again. He didn't care. He was in enormous pain
from his hand and head and neck, but that was nothing com-
pared with the anguish of every conscious moment. He was
desperate to sleep, to retreat into a place where he didn't have
to know or remember. But sleep eluded him and in the darkness each night he was left alone with the pain that assaulted
him on all fronts. When he finally did fall asleep, it was with
the hope that the morning might not come. So he didn't care
what hope the doctors thought they could offer. He didn't want
to move. He didn't want to live.

When he arrived at the TRI, he was as depressed as he'd
ever been. Despite the profound love he had for his children
and his desire to still be a good father, he simply could not
dredge up the will to go on. It was too hard, he couldn't do it,
the pain was too deep and too cruel. Please, he just wanted to
sleep, oh God, please let him sleep.

When he opened his eyes, something was different. There
was a man sitting beside his bed, looking straight at him. Stan
looked back, blankly. He knew he ought to be wondering who
this guy was, but he couldn't bring himself to be curious.

"Stan. I've been waiting for you. We've never met, but I
know all about you. I'm Howard—Howard Rocket. We've both
got challenges here, let's meet them, what do you say?"

Stan looked at this visitor more closely. Howard Rocket.
Stan knew about him, too. Howard's sister, Tyrral, had been

Susan's golf partner. He'd known all about his stroke, about how he'd defied the odds and survived surgery. He guessed that was how Howard knew about him. Stan appreciated the gesture, but didn't have the strength to make friends right now. He hoped Howard would leave soon.

But Howard continued talking. "... you're mobile and I'm not, but I can move these wheels. You can move your legs, there's no reason for you to be in a hospital bed all day. Let's go for a walk, I'll give you the tour."

Stan found himself focusing on what Howard was saying. He had to focus, Howard was speaking so quickly. *Get up, get going, you can do it, come on*—this man was remarkable, to be such a cheerleader after what he himself had gone through. Stan didn't know why Howard seemed to care so much about whether or not he got out of bed, especially when he himself didn't. But he appreciated the effort, futile though it was. Stan just wanted to sleep.

But Howard just wanted to help, and was convinced that he could. He saw in Stan the rock-bottom helplessness that he himself had pushed away before it had had time to settle around his heart. Howard feared for this man who didn't seem to want to exist. He wanted to help reawaken his will to live. He wouldn't stop until he had succeeded.

Stan had a long way to go, but Howard had all the time in the world. He sat with Stan for hours and hours, talking away about everything that passed through his head, letting his energy surround them both. They were strangers, but they had something very deep in common. Howard exhorted and encouraged Stan to get out of bed; and finally—he did. Stan didn't know what it was that made him decide to accompany this man on his stroll down the hallway, but suddenly he realized that he would ... like that.

They'd go up and down the hall, Stan on foot and Howard

on wheels, and they would talk. Much of the time Howard would lead the conversation, and Stan would listen, marvelling at how a stranger could be so frank about so much. Howard talked about his family with excitement and joy, and Stan would think about his own wonderful children, Dana and Jon, and how much they meant to him, and what a wonderful reason to live they were.

He didn't know whether it was his kids or Howard or simply the passage of time, but he began to get better. He went to therapy and his hand started to get better. His memory returned, and so did his appreciation of life. Every day he would sit with Howard and talk, or he'd let Howard do the talking and he'd take something from that.

He kept Howard's messages when he was finally released from the hospital. He had two wonderful children to come home to, and he was still alive. He had pain that would never go away, and moments of anguish so bitter that he couldn't imagine living through them, but at the end of it all he still had something in him that was able to face another day. Life went on. And, with a little help from Howard, he actually wanted to live it.

By mid-January Howard had outgrown the Toronto Rehabilitation Institute. He was healthy now, stable, and mobile. He'd already been spending extended periods of time at home, and now felt ready to return for good. He knew he wouldn't be confined to the ground floor for long. His physio and occupational therapists had sent him along with their blessings. Most important, Glenda had given her approval. She knew it was time for her patient to leave. He was ready, even if she wasn't sure she was.

Dr. Jim Ruderman, the physician supervising Howard's case at the TRI, approved Howard's discharge, and met with the family and a social worker to explain where the healing process would proceed from that point. They learned how to apply for Wheel-Trans so that Howard might travel easily and comfortably in his wheelchair; who to speak with concerning outpatient therapy; how often to book follow-up appointments to assess his blood content and ensure that he maintained correct balance. These were the new rules guiding a new stage in his life. Howard couldn't wait to get on with it.

They were more cautious now than they had been, and their optimism was tempered with the knowledge that problems could still develop. They had all been euphoric about Howard's progress and the leaps and bounds he was making. There had been no indication that anything would hold him back now. But there had been something. Another clot, this time in a vein. A few weeks into his stay at the TRI, Howard had begun to notice a pain in his left leg. He had been at home when he'd first become conscious of it, and he told Debbie. She had examined his leg and even her untrained eye could tell that it was swollen. *Oh, God, not again.* Fighting her rising fear, she put him in the car and returned to the Toronto Western. How familiar this emergency room was. How she had hoped that she'd never see it again.

They had run a "doppler" on Howard—a test that scanned for clots. Sure enough, the doppler showed a DVT— deep vein thrombosis. A vein this time. Not as serious a clot, but a clot nonetheless. Howard seemed to be somewhat susceptible. Clearly, they had something to worry about.

Howard was furious. Here he was, doing so well, trying so hard, and wham! He got knocked down just when he was pulling himself up. For the first time, the words *it's not fair* crossed his brain, despite his efforts not to feel sorry for himself. But it was hard, dammit. Now he had to wait for this clot to be dissolved before he could resume physiotherapy, and he knew that his muscle memory wouldn't last long. But there was nothing he could do except take his blood-thinning medication and hope for the best.

As before, he'd been lucky. The clot responded well to the medication, and the thrombosis subsided. Now that the doctors were aware of the possibility of clotting, his blood was more closely regulated and examined. They had him wearing anti-embolic stockings, and Dana would crack up looking at him, propped up in bed with those thick beige tights on, applying pressure on his legs to avoid pooling of blood.

It wasn't as if Howard had been taking his new-found health for granted prior to this setback, but now he was even more aware that anything could happen. Returning home was progress, but it was also risky; there were no nurses or doctors to scurry to his side when called. Independence was a function of getting better, but it was a little scary, too. Nevertheless, Howard knew that he was ready, risks or not. And home was where he belonged.

He'd been home now for almost ten months, riding the healing process with his family. He'd made all the big leaps by that time, and turned his attention to the smaller challenges of his situation. He still attended therapy twice a week at Toronto Rehabilitation Centre, an outpatient facility. He loved his therapy, and would not sacrifice a second of it despite the demands of his daily work. Business had its place now. Howard still loved it, still loved turning his mind to new problems and finding new solutions, but there were other things that came first. Health, and family, and friends, and self. It was all part of the healing process that never quite stopped, however healthy you were.

He would drive himself now to rehab sessions—a far cry from his first visit. The Wheel-Trans bus had been booked and had come to pick him up at home. He'd felt like a kid on his way to school, which he supposed he was. Dana, Amie, and Debbie had stood at the door, watching him go and waving to him as he drove away. He found out later that Dana had waited a few minutes and then followed him in her car, feeling like an idiot but wanting to be sure he was all right. Talk about role reversal.

Howard loved rehab for several reasons. Of course he loved the exercise and the push and the raw physical feeling of overcoming an obstacle. He could feel the difference in his muscles every time, steadily and surely. He worked with Bev Jones, his physiotherapist, and Cecile McKennit, his occupational therapist. Bev focused with Howard on his gross movements and how he could control his body, showing him how the right way to move was supposed to feel, so he could learn that feeling and recreate it at home, until that movement and that feeling became instinctive. Howard worked hard with Bev, eager to please and eager to achieve, pushing and pushing and pushing some more, and she'd laugh at Howard's aggressive strides and his driving need to get there *now*, and guide him in the right direction. Cecile took what Howard had learned with Bev and taught Howard to apply it to his everyday movements, like turning a key or tying shoelaces. All simple tasks that were Howard's daily challenges.

By now those challenges were fewer. He'd left the wheelchair behind for good in April, using a cane for balance but not needing a whole lot else. The family removed the ramps, lowered the table, and returned the Rocket living room to its previous state. Howard had moved upstairs, returning to the bedroom he hadn't seen since that day long ago when he'd dialed 911 from his bedside. The house was once again his. Welcome home, Howard.

Now, again, the family was all together under one roof. Amie had long since finished her degree and was working at a brokerage house in downtown Toronto. She was learning the ropes and gaining valuable experience that she could eventually take to a business partnership with her eager dad. Howard couldn't wait to work with his daughter.

Dana was his constant companion, if not in person then on the cellular phone. She still nursed fears that wouldn't quite let go, but she had finally accepted that it was impossible to protect him forever, that Howard had to do his own thing and go his own way and take whatever risks came with that. But she would take care of him as much as she could for as long as she could, and that made her happy.

The extended family was still as tightly knit as ever, thanks to that October day a year ago. Now they didn't wait for seders and bat mitzvahs as reason to see each other; getting together was reason enough. Back at the New Year's party they came up with the idea of drawing up a definitive schedule of planned family events, each member alternating in the role of host. Since then the schedule held as planned, through holidays and just for good times. The Rockets had hosted a Mother's Day brunch up at their cottage, and the day had been beautiful with plenty of sunshine and exhilaration. The kids had been running around and the adults had been chasing them and laughing together. Howard had bought a golf cart and zoomed around with different nieces in tow, yelling in delight along with them.

He had also got into the habit of lunching weekly with his sisters. The contact felt really good after all these years—of course the connections were always intact but it was refreshing to experience them on a regular basis. Each took turns choosing a restaurant and driving the others there, although Howard ended up doing most of the driving because he loved it so much. He was glad to be able to drive now, he still remembered being picked up by his sisters while he was still in the wheelchair— they hadn't been very adept at helping their brother into the chair at the beginning, and they'd all had a whole lot of laughter over their clumsy attempts to haul him from the car and into the chair. They'd eventually learned the hard way, and it had been fine, but Howard was quite happy to be doing the driving now.

They'd be having another get-together in the not-so-distant future. One of the happiest moments of his life was scheduled for the coming May: Amie and Michael were going to be married. With familiar, strong emotion, he recalled that day in December when Michael had asked for his daughter's hand. He'd been at home for a weekend, enjoying the quiet of the afternoon. Both Amie and Dana had been out. He'd heard the dogs barking wildly, and heard Debbie answer the door, heard Michael's familiar voice, had been pleased. Michael was very special to him, in fact both Michaels were. He had a relationship with them both that was independent of his daughters. Howard considered them both friends, on par with Michael Winton or Brian Price. Michael Wuls had all but left school during Howard's illness, had thrown everything up to fly halfway around the world for his daughter, had patiently fed spoonful after spoonful of hospital food into his mouth for God knows how many meals, and had helped look after the mundane details of life in order to release Debbie from that burden. He was always glad to see him.

Michael had walked into the living room and had sat by Howard's bed, leaning in close. He'd taken Howard's hand and said simply, "Howard, I want to marry your daughter. I want you to be my best man, and I want you to walk down the aisle at our wedding." And Howard, for whom speaking had never been a challenge, could only nod with emotion, tears welling in his eyes, and hold Michael's hands even tighter.

Michael's eyes, too, were moist. "I'm coming to you first with this because Amie is your daughter and your blessing is important to me. I also want you to know that I'm prepared to wait, if you want me to." He looked at Howard expectantly.

Howard was overcome. His voice was hoarse. "I want you to do it right away. And I will walk down that aisle." Then they were both laughing and hugging, and Debbie ran in and soon she was laughing and hugging too, and Michael was laughing because he'd loved Amie so much for so long and he'd been wanting to propose for some time, but she'd been in Tokyo and then her father had been ill and he'd told himself that he ought to wait and now he finally didn't have to wait anymore and he could spend the rest of his life with the woman he adored.

◆　◆　◆

Now, one year later, Howard reflected on how lucky he was. Truly, he was blessed with the most wonderful things in life, the important things, and he was doubly blessed because now he was able to appreciate how lucky he was. Knowing all that he knew now, about the pain and the struggle and the frustration and the fear, and about the joy and the triumph and the sweetness and the love, he would do it all again without changing a moment. For him the last year had been the product of a single, profound stroke of luck, a great gift that showed itself over and over in the many, many gifts that surrounded him each day. He had his health, finally, and although he would never have all the capabilities he once had, he had never felt better, nor more alive. He had family, surrounding him with love: his mother and his sisters and his children and his wife, and his nieces and their children in a great circle of love that flowed through them all and was bound together by their hearts. He had his friends who, through steadfast support and understanding, had demonstrated what loyalty and caring could mean and to what lengths they could be taken. And he had his work, in which he continued to find daily fulfillment and challenge.

Howard had learned some of the hardest lessons through his work, lessons that weren't about his inability to move his leg or swing his nephew in his arms. These were emotional lessons about the flip side of the coin, which he'd caught more than a glimpse of during this whole struggle. Business dealings were complex under normal circumstances, but his stroke had thrown a new set of challenges into the equation. He had thought that business partners were just that: partners—people who worked together with him as a unit. Well, he'd had some surprises in that area, some betrayals that shocked and hurt. And it wasn't so much the money or the power in the transaction, it was the knowledge that, for some, tolerance and support and loyalty came second to self-interest and fear.

But he'd turned the difficult lessons of those betrayals into a part of the healing process, recognizing that it was far more important to identify those for whom the relationships ran deep than to lament the departure of those preoccupied with their own interests. And he hadn't allowed the difficulties he'd encountered to affect his ambition or goals. Howard was still driven by the motivation to succeed, and refused to be dragged down by personal disappointments or financial setbacks. He'd been through a lot worse, and he hadn't been beaten. He never let himself forget that.

Now he was complete again, perhaps for the first time. He had everything important that a man could ever want or need, had been blessed a thousand times over with good fortune and good friends and good luck, which he knew by now was the most important blessing of all. He knew now the importance of the little things that he once could do and took for granted, and that once he couldn't do and yearned to achieve. Now that he could do them again, he was grateful and he was proud and he was humbled and he was aware. Now he could take a shower, take a step, take a breath, and every time he did, he remembered how lucky he was and how each one was to be treasured. Because taking a shower meant more than cleansing, taking a step meant more than moving, taking a breath meant more than breathing. They meant freedom, they meant joy, they meant humanity, they meant love.

They meant life.

Life

Howard stood in place behind the closed doors. Beyond those doors was a room filled with people he loved, who loved him, who loved his family, who were part of their lives. They had gathered to celebrate life together on one of the most amazing days Howard had ever known. Again, tears filled his eyes. Debbie's hand was in his own, the reassuring warmth of her grip calming and exhilarating at the same time. He looked at his beautiful wife, with whom he had shared so much over the years. They were about to share another wonderful experience, another sweet moment in a life filled with such moments.

He could hear the murmuring from behind the doors stop suddenly, and realized they had opened. The first members of the procession were slowly walking through them as the music began. A sea of faces turned toward the doors, with smiles and some tears, but only of happiness. Flowers seemed to be everywhere. Debbie's grip grew tighter. His own had as well.

Howard had left his cane behind. He had no desire to use it, no need. He was about to fulfill a promise made over a year ago. There was no place for a cane in that promise.

Suddenly he was looking directly at all the faces. The procession had moved forward, and it was their turn now. Debbie held him firmly, reassuring him with her strength and her warmth. She was there for him, as always, and this was just another step that they would take together. Howard took a breath, and began to walk.

He focused on different faces in the audience as he moved, with some stiffness but no difficulty. He'd walked now for quite some time, but no journey had ever seemed quite as important as this one. He looked ahead toward the *chupah*, under which stood the man who was about to marry his daughter, the man who would become his son. He was walking down the aisle at Michael and Amie's wedding, as promised.

Then they were there, at the front, standing together with Michael's parents and the groom, and Howard could breathe again and watch the procession continue. There were his tiny nephews and nieces, walking carefully in time down the aisle, giggling and glowing with the importance of their role. There was his daughter Dana, beaming so beautifully, walking with grace and confidence and exuberance down the aisle, holding her flowers before her like a promise. She arrived and stood with her parents, giving her father's hand a quick squeeze before turning her attention to the final member of the procession.

There really were no words to describe that emotion, watching one's daughter take the measured walk from youth to womanhood, from child to adult, from her family's house to her own family. Amie moved so beautifully down that aisle, looking breathtakingly beautiful as only a bride could look. But this was a special bride. His daughter. Her wedding. Her life.

Afterward, at the reception, he realized how important that moment was to him. He had experienced such profound emotion on a few occasions in his life, many years ago at his own wedding, upon the birth of his daughters, and upon his own birth, his rebirth, just a scant year and a half ago. He realized how close he had come to not being there, leaving behind an empty seat at the head table, a solemn pause during the speeches and an ache in the hearts that would have missed him so much at this moment. Now that he was here, he planned to make the most of this wonderful evening, as he now made the most of every moment of his life.

This was one of the rites of his family's intertwined lives. They'd grown up together over two decades, four people joined by love. The bonds were not changing, but the units of measurement were. They were still a family, but they were not the only family. And that was good, so very, very good.

Howard had made himself a promise many years ago when Amie was born, and tonight was the night it would be realized. They had eaten, and danced, and laughed together much over the course of that evening, but he had not yet voiced his emotion. And there was much he wanted to say. It was time.

Slowly, the clinking of glasses and the murmuring of voices was stilled, as everyone assembled turned their attention to Howard. Each person there knew what had happened a year and a half ago. It was a knowledge that charged the air, an awareness that deepened the celebration. Howard had their full attention.

"I'm going to turn your attention over here, away from the head table to the dance floor. Amie, Michael, come over here." He motioned them over to the stage and into two chairs, one on either side of him. He started walking, and they followed him. He was using his cane.

"As most of you know, I had a stroke a year and a half ago. Many of you were there for me and my family and know how close I was to not being here today. Well, I'm here and I'm not going anywhere, you can bet on that." Laughter, and anticipation. "But I'm not going to talk about what happened a year and a half ago. It happened, I'm better, and I have a wonderful life. I want to talk about something that happened almost twenty-five years ago. I had a beautiful wife, Debbie, and we were expecting a beautiful baby. Well, we got one. Amie." He paused to look at her, and smiled. She smiled back.

"And I made a promise to myself on that day. I promised that I would dance with my daughter at her wedding. And I had a song picked out, and I knew I would dance with my beautiful daughter at some time in the future, to that song. She was about five minutes old at that time.

"Well, a year and a half ago I had a stroke. And for a long time, I couldn't walk, and I couldn't move, and I couldn't do a lot of things. But I've worked hard and I've been lucky, and I can do most of those things now. But I haven't yet danced. I've been waiting, for this moment." He motioned to the band, and the first few bars of music began.

"Now, I'm going to fulfill that promise, and I'm going to dance with my daughter on her wedding day." And he stood up, and handed his cane to Michael. And he reached out his other hand to his daughter, who took it, her eyes moist. And there, in the center of the floor, they began to dance.

Howard could hear his friends and family applauding as he turned slowly in the middle of the dance floor, his eyes moving around the room across the faces of the guests. Friends from so long ago, Shelly Little from his childhood and Lorne Frohman from his youth and Brian Price from his early days in business. There were his sisters and his mother and his nieces, some with children of their own, and Michael's family, his parents and his sister with her own husband and child, all smiling into the center of the ballroom where a father held his daughter in his arms on her wedding day.

He held his daughter, of whom he was so very proud. She was so worthy of being loved so much, and she had found someone who could love her completely and wholly and utterly, who had stood before them all and had pledged to adore her for the rest of his life, and she had done the same. There were so many blessings in this room, so many gifts.

He could see Debbie and Dana watching them, and smiled at both of them. They were his everything, his family, his life. He looked at his daughter, and then he looked at his new son-in-law, still holding his cane, and was happy to share. He gently turned from his daughter, and motioned Michael over. And he took back his cane as he gave back his daughter, and moved to the side to watch them dance together as husband and wife.

And as they moved together on the dance floor, Howard took his wife in his arms and led her out, and Michael's parents came too, and Dana and her own Michael, and slowly the dance floor filled up around the bride and groom, each couple a circle of love that joined in circling them with love.

Howard felt very much a part of that circle, felt strongly the power of emotion and devotion that linked each of these people together in a lifetime connection. He'd felt it in the ICU, had known that each stone that was dropped into a pool sent out ripples in every direction, and that those ripples were a part of that stone just as surely as the stone was the reason for the ripples, or else that stone would simply drop to the bottom without having any impact at all. And Howard finally knew that that was what life was about, it was about having an impact on those you love, being their ripples and they being yours, interacting with them to make their lives better and fuller and more complete, and by doing so fulfilling your own. And his life felt complete in that room, with all of his ripples collected in one place, flowing into the stone instead of away from it.

And again, as he had done so many times before and as he would forever into the future, Howard was grateful.

He had such wonderful, wonderful luck.

Epilogue

A nd that's my story. The story of a guy lucky enough to have two lives—one to learn from, and one to live right. Most people don't have that chance. Most people don't have that luck.

Most people would be glad not to. Lying on your back in an ICU with tubes weaving through your body isn't anybody's idea of a good time. But it was a small price to pay, considering all I got in return.

You're lucky. You don't have to go through it to learn what I've learned. You don't have to suffer a stroke to know what I know. This book just told you. And if you found yourself moved by even one word in it, then I've shown you something. If I started you thinking, even for a moment, then I've been the blackboard, the billboard, the flashing light that I wanted to be. I hope the lesson has sunk in. Learning the hard way is one tough road.

But it's a road that anyone can travel, really. I said before that I'm not unique, and I truly believe that. I'm just a guy who had a hell of a lot to live for, a hell of a lot of good reasons to fight. And struggling toward life isn't really a struggle, especially considering the alternative.

It's an interesting road to travel, really, because it never quite ends. Sure, I've pretty much reached my plateau. I know I'll probably never be capable of all I once was. So what? That gives me something to strive for. They said I wouldn't move, they said I wouldn't walk. Well, I walked down the aisle at my daughter's wedding. I danced with her, sure and upright and confident. There couldn't be a better reason to keep on striving than that.

Motivation like that kept me from melting into the darkness, when I felt myself falling and the light beckoned. There were so many reasons to come back. Family. Friends. Love. I couldn't leave my daughters, not when we had so much more to give each other. And I know I was right to come back, because I got to dance at Amie's wedding and soon I'll be walking down the aisle at Dana's. What else is there to live for, really? For a father to witness the joy of his children is the purest, most real blessing possible. These were the gifts worth fighting for.

I've learned to love this fight. Every day there are new goals to set, old accomplishments to build on. They said I wouldn't walk, but I've taught myself to run again. Left foot, right foot. Left foot, right foot. The steps I take are easier now but I haven't forgotten. And every time I remember, I push harder, until the steps come easier and until they come faster. And then one day I was able to raise my knees enough to lift one foot off the ground while the other pushed off, hard. And then I was running.

And they said I wouldn't even walk.

I ran for half a mile. Then I had to stop. I couldn't do any more, not then. But I know how to run now, and I'll keep going and push it up to three-quarters, and then I'll break a mile, and then I'll keep going. I'm not worried about when it will happen; I know that it will.

So where does this leave us? I know who I am, and where I'm going, and what I need. Do you? I've learned my lesson, discovered what's important. Have you? I love, I am loved. Are you?

I know now that each stone dropped into a pool sends out ripples in all directions, and those ripples are a part of that stone just as surely as the stone was the reason for the ripples, or else that stone would simply drop to the bottom without having any impact at all.

And that's what life is about, it's about having an impact on those you love, being their ripples and they being yours, interacting with them to make their lives better and fuller and more complete, and by so doing, your own. And I'm lucky, because my ripples flow into the stone, too.

And really, that's the story.

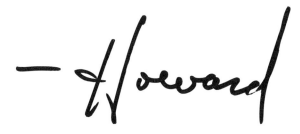

Fears & Prayers

I cry because you're suffering,
Each night I shed a tear.
I cry because my heart aches,
I wish that you were near.

I pray because I worry,
Although I know you're well.
I pray because I love you,
Even more than words can tell.

I cry because I miss you,
I think about you every day.
I cry because I'm very proud,
That you came such a long way.

I pray because I'm a believer,
I know you will be fine.
I pray because I'm grateful,
That through the darkness light did shine.

I've shed so many tears,
And my prayers have been long.
Uncle Howie don't lose your faith,
You're a fighter and you're strong.

Uncle Howie I must tell you,
In my life you play a special part.
Most importantly you must realize,
That you have really touched my heart.

I Love You,
Love, Lauren

—Lauren Baker is the 12-year-old daughter of Howard's sister, Marsha, and her husband Shelly.

Resources and Support

A guide to stroke information, support groups, agencies, and web sites

National Resource Organizations

U.S. Department of Health & Human Services
Public Health Service—Agency for Health Care Policy
& Research
P.O. Box 8547
Silver Spring, MD   20907-8547
800-358-9295
Governmental publications are available on a variety of stroke related topics, including the widely acclaimed Post-Stroke Rehabilitation Clinical Practice Guidelines *and* Recovering After a Stroke: Post-Stroke Rehabilitation Patient and Family Guide.

American Heart Association
Stroke Connection
7272 Greenville Avenue
Dallas, TX   75231
800-553-5321
Toll-free referral and information for stroke survivors, caregivers, family members and health care professionals. Stroke Connection also offers free stroke materials, National Stroke Support Group Registry, Stroke Peer Visitor Programs, and Stroke Connection Magazine, *the premier voice on stroke, for stroke audiences.*

American Association of Retired Persons (AARP)
601 E Street, NW
Washington, DC   20049
800-424-2277
This organization provides information relating to aging and senior citizens. They also have literature for a variety of health and benefit questions for seniors.

Survivor and Rehabilitation Resources

American Academy of Physical Medicine and Rehabilitation
1 IBM Plaza, Suite 2500
Chicago, IL   60611
312-464-9700
This is an automated information line that provides listings of physiatrists in local areas.

American Occupational Therapy Association
4720 Montgomery Lane
Bethesda, MD   20814
301-652-2682
This association helps people locate occupational therapists in their local areas.

American Physical Therapy Association
1111 North Fairfax Street
Alexandria, VA   22314
703-684-2782
This national organization provides referrals to state chapters.

American Speech-Language-Hearing Association
10801 Rockville Pike
Rockville, MD   20852
800-638-8255 or 301-498-2071
This organization can provide a list of speech therapists in your state.

National Aphasia Association
40 East 34th Street, Room RR 306
New York, NY   10016
800-922-4622
This organization provides information and support services for people living with aphasia.

National Association of Social Workers
750 1st Street, NE
Washington, DC   20002
202-408-8600 or 800-638-8799
This national association provides a list of local social workers.

National Easter Seal Society
230 West Monroe Street, Suite 1800
Chicago, IL   60606
800-221-6827
This organization helps people with disabilities achieve independence by locating funding sources to assist with medical/assistive equipment and medical bills (on occasion).

National Institute of Neurological Disorders and Stroke
9000 Rockville Pike, Building 31, Room 8A-16
Bethesda, MD   20892
800-352-9424
This organization receives funding from the National Institute of Health and provides clinical information packets on stroke.

National Rehabilitation Information Center
8455 Colesville Road, Suite 935
Silver Spring, MD   20910-3319
800-346-2742
This toll-free number provides information on types of rehabilitation, adaptive devices and other aids for recovery.

Vocational Services for the Disabled
800-222-JOBS
A New York-based service that refers consumers to local state offices providing vocational and educational services for individuals with disabilities.

Caregiver Resources

Eldercare Locator
1112 16th Street NW, Suite 100
Washington, DC   20036
800-677-1116
A nationwide database that gives caregivers access to local areas' resources that provide care to the elderly.

Family Caregiver Alliance
425 Bush Street, Suite 500
San Francisco, CA   94108
415-434-3388 or 800-445-8106 in California
This organization provides caregiver support and educational opportunities through research, advocacy, legal consultation and training workshops.

National Council on Aging
409 Third Street, SW, Second Floor
Washington, DC   20024
800-375-1014
This organization provides lists of community resources that help improve the quality of life for the elderly.

Flying Wheels Travel
143 West Bridge Street
Owatonna, MN   55060
800-535-6790
This agency provides worldwide travel assistance for the disabled.

Mental Health Resources

American Association of Suicidology
4202 Connecticut Avenue, Suite 310
Washington, DC   20008
202-237-2280
This association provides information on suicide and a referral to the nearest suicide crisis center in your area.

American Psychiatric Association
1400 K Street, NW
Washington, DC   20005
202-682-6000
This organization provides information on choosing a psychiatrist as well as research on emotional illness.

Depression Awareness, Recognition and Treatment (D/ART)
National Institute of Mental Health
5600 Fishers Lane
Rockville, MD   20857
800-421-4211
This organization is an educational resource for the general public as well as health care professionals on the co-occurrence of stroke and depression.

National Foundation for Depressive Illness
P.O. Box 2257
New York, NY   10116
800-239-1265
This foundation provides information and referrals to the public about depressive illnesses.

Financial Resources

Medicare Hotline
P.O. Box 50463
Indianapolis, IN   46250-0463
800-638-6833
Call this toll-free number for information about Medicare and financial assistance for persons over 65. They can also help find medical specialists in local areas.

Social Security
P.O. Box 1756
Baltimore, MD   21235
800-772-1213
A national toll-free number that provides assistance with Social Security benefit questions, and makes referrals to local Social Security offices.

National Insurance Consumer Helpline
110 William Street
New York, NY   10038
800-942-4242
This toll-free number provides assistance with questions about health/ life insurance as well as information about individual health insurance companies.

Patient Rights Resources

People's Medical Society
462 Walnut Street
Allentown, PA   18102
610-770-1670
This organization provides information designed to make every American a smart health care consumer.

Employment Resources

ADA Helpline—Equal Employment Opportunity Commission
P.O. Box 12549
Cincinnati, OH   45212-0549
800-669-4000
This is a toll-free number for information about discrimination against people with disabilities in the workforce.

Higher Education & Training for People with Handicaps
800-544-3284
This is an automated information line that provides information on post-secondary education for the disabled.

IBM's National Support Center for Persons with Disabilities
800-426-4832
This center serves as a clearinghouse to help health care leaders, agency directors, policy makers, employers, educators, public officials and individuals learn how computers can enhance the quality of life in the school, home and workplace for persons with disabilities.

Internet Web Sites

Howard Rocket's book, *A Stroke of Luck*, maintains a special web site that features a discussion group, recorded audio commentary by Dr. Rocket, and a complete media kit: Check it out at http://www.StrokeOfLuck.com/

- National Stroke Association
  http://www.stroke.org/

- American Heart and Stroke Association
  http://www.amhrt.org/catalog/Stroke_catpage30.html

- WholeNurse Stroke Information
  http://www.wholenurse.com/stroke.htm

- The Brain Matters Stroke Initiative
  http://www.strokematters.com/

- The Stanford University Stroke Center
  http://www.med.stanford.edu/school/stroke/

- Mayo Clinic Stroke Education
  http://www.mayo.edu/cerebro/education/stroke.html

- American Academy of Neurology - Stroke Fact Sheet
  http://www.aan.com/public/stro.html

- Stroke WebForum at Massachusetts General Hospital
  http://neuro-www.mgh.harvard.edu/forum/StrokeMenu.html

Writer's Postscript

Not many writers my age are given an opportunity like this. Writing this book has been a challenge, and a learning experience, and a stroke of luck in its own right.

This project was almost two years in the making, and during that time I received support and assistance from many people. Chief among them were my parents, whose editorial contributions, frank assessments, and constant encouragement made the finished product that much better. I also owe a debt to Johnny Connon, whose red penstrokes across my rough drafts gave me the objectivity I needed to do this project justice.

Finally, I am grateful to Howard Rocket and his family for opening their lives and trusting me to tell their story. It is a story I am glad to have witnessed, and chronicled, and shared.

—Rachel Sklar
November 24, 1997

Final Thoughts from the Publisher

Ifirst met Howard Rocket in March, 1988. I was waiting in the 25th floor office lobby of Tridont Health Care Inc., about to sign some papers to join the company as number-two person in corporate communications. Howard Rocket, the company chairman, strode confidently to the front receptionist, asking for his messages. He looked up, flashed his perfect smile and said, "Hi there."

For the next several years I worked hand-in-hand with Howard, through all the ups and downs of that great enterprise called Tridont. Then we lost touch until a law firm seminar one morning in September, 1996.

Is that Howard Rocket? At first sight I honestly could not tell for certain. The cane, the hesitant gait, the limp arm, the loss of weight. Is that really him? I asked a colleague. "Yes, of course, that's Howard Rocket; he had a stroke last October, you know."

I could not believe what I was hearing. A stroke. That only happens to old people, or so I had thought. I sat next to him at the lecture. He asked me to hold his cane for a moment. I was still unsure what to say. Howard did the talking for me. "I want to publish a book about this experience; can you help?"

With that invitation another chapter in Howard's life was about to be opened: Howard Rocket, book author. Under the creative guidance of Rachel Sklar, a capable and energetic writer, the manuscript took solid form through fall and winter 1996, then spring and summer 1997.

We tapped Howard's extensive network of associates and the effort really took flight. The Toronto Rehabilitation Institute Foundation stepped forward as beneficiary of the project. Howard had spent the most challenging months of his life at TRI, one of North America's leading treatment and rehabilitation centers for stroke survivors. Without the care of the entire staff at TRI , Howard Rocket would not be what he is today: capable, successful, spirited, and 98% physically recovered.

To support this book we have established a state-of-the-art web site and online discussion area that we hope will facilitate exchange of views and supportive messages among stroke survivors and their families in Canada, USA, and around the world. We invite you to check it out and contribute your responses: *http://www.StrokeOfLuck.com/*

I hope you have enjoyed reading this book as much as Howard, Rachel, and our production team enjoyed making it. There is deeper meaning within these pages, and we hope you will find it.

—William C. Stratas
president@planetcast.com
November 26, 1997